Liver

Detox

Natural Liver Detox Providing Liver Aid While Restoring Liver Health

(The Ultimate Cleansing Program for Long-term Liver Health)

John Ellis

Published By **Oliver Leish**

John Ellis

All Rights Reserved

Liver Detox: Natural Liver Detox Providing Liver Aid While Restoring Liver Health (The Ultimate Cleansing Program for Long-term Liver Health)

ISBN   978-1-998927-98-2

No part of this guidebook shall be reproduced in any form without permission in writing from the publisher except in the case of brief quotations embodied in critical articles or reviews.

Legal & Disclaimer

The information contained in this book is not designed to replace or take the place of any form of medicine or professional medical advice. The information in this book has been provided for educational & entertainment purposes only.

The information contained in this book has been compiled from sources deemed reliable, and it is accurate to the best of the Author's knowledge; however, the Author cannot guarantee its accuracy and validity and cannot be held liable for any errors or omissions. Changes are periodically made to this book. You must consult your doctor or get professional medical advice before using any of the suggested remedies, techniques, or information in this book.

Table Of Contents

Chapter 1: Know Your Liver

Before you could apprehend what it's far that a liver detox can do for you, you'll need a better information of what your liver is and why it's far essential for your survival and health. This first bankruptcy will cowl the whole lot you need to understand about the liver and its function and a way to recognize if a liver detox is proper for you.

Please endure in thoughts that each one vital organs to your body need to be cared for in ways unique to their functionality. The purpose of this ebook is to talk approximately the liver mainly and how a liver detox and manner of lifestyles changes can enhance your everyday health as regards to your liver. If you've got have been given concerns approximately the opportunity organs for your frame, you may likely discover that starting together along with your liver allows to treatment some of the issues that have led you to be concerned about the opportunity organs.

With that during mind, permit's get proper into the liver!

Introduction to the Liver

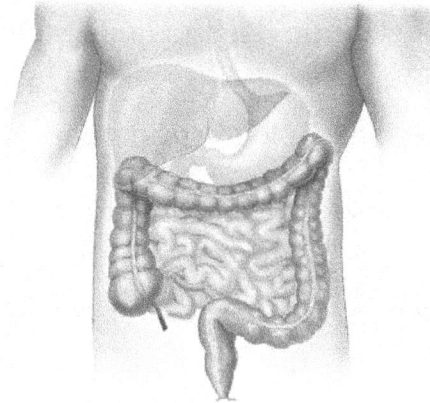

Making up sort of 2% of an character's frame weight, the liver is the most vital internal human organ. The liver sits on the right aspect of the abdominopelvic body hollow space, above the small and massive gut, barely overlapping the belly. The liver is essential because it helps many body structures, which includes the immune gadget, digestive device, and other metabolic techniques. In truth, the liver has a characteristic in nearly every organ device inside the body, collectively with the endocrine device and the gastrointestinal systems.

In wellknown, the liver is liable for maintaining the blood clean, casting off toxins from the blood, metabolizing sex hormones and precise metabolic skills, and producing company proteins that make contributions to replicate and improvement. The liver isn't only a filtration organ, even though. It additionally stores crucial minerals and vitamins, like iron and copper. It moreover plays an essential function in cholesterol regulation.

The liver is a totally unique organ in that it has extraordinary regenerative residences. If someone desires a liver transplant, every now and then, they'll be capable of get a dwelling donor transplant. What this means is that a matching donor can donate a lobe in their liver to the affected individual in want of a transplant. After the lobe is well implanted into the patient and their vintage liver is eliminated, the lobe can expand to a entire, functioning length in only a few weeks. The donor doesn't lose the capability in their liver each because of the fact the organ regenerates the lobe that end up eliminated.

Knowing approximately the liver's regenerative homes makes it possible to understand that an overtaxed liver or a partially damaged liver has the ability to heal and regenerate itself if given the possibility.

The Liver's Primary Function

As you may have discerned from the previous phase, the liver has masses of particular capabilities in the body. This section goes to interrupt down the full-size array of abilties into the primary capabilities of the liver and their significance. Having a better knowledge of what your liver does inner your frame will with a piece of luck assist you to look why the liver needs to be looked after.

Bile Production

The kidneys are a waste elimination organ inside the frame. However, not all wastes can be removed by using the use of the usage of the kidneys. This is wherein bile is available in. One of the bile's primary abilities is to excrete cloth that isn't removed via the kidneys. Bile additionally performs an essential position in the absorption of lipids inside the body. Bile is an vital substance on the subject of doing away with waste within the frame and also preserving intestine, gut, and bowel health.

The liver is the organ that produces this important bodily substance. Bile isn't truly created inside the liver; it's also recycled yet again to the liver. Through this production and recycle machine, the liver allows to create a substance the body desires after which removes the waste once it is used. It makes a closed system, but that device wants to be kept wholesome to paintings.

If the gut and bowel aren't at pinnacle-nice health, the body can begin to revel in a lot of problems, in conjunction with irritable bowel syndrome, inflammatory bowel illness, and bile malabsorption. If bile isn't produced nicely or recycled by means of manner of the liver, the whole gastrointestinal and digestive tool may be thrown right into a nation of illness and malfunction.

Fat-Soluble Vitamin Storage/Metabolism

The human body requires a stability of numerous vitamins to hold health and well-being. Common vitamins that humans apprehend approximately, typically because of a deficiency, are nutrients A, B, C, D, E, and K. There are many different vitamins that the human frame dreams, despite the truth that.

Most nutrients can be fed on via meals and with a wholesome, balanced eating regimen. Others are taken in from the surroundings, like vitamins D, which can be absorbed through the eyes and skin from publicity to daytime. If you've ever professional a nutrition deficiency, you can had been recommended by way of using a physician or fitness care company to take a dietary complement that has focused quantities of the vitamins you want more of. Whether it is through diet, dietary supplements, or environmental factors, vitamins are taken into the frame and are answerable for some of one-of-a-type chemical and bodily procedures in the body.

Vitamins A, D, E, and K are referred to as fats-soluble nutrients. This technique that they're all soluble in natural solvents. They are also metabolized, transported, and absorbed in a similar manner as fat. These fats-soluble nutrients are people who the liver in the end finally ends up being liable for.

Most fat-soluble vitamins tour to the liver from the intestines, wherein they may be absorbed. Once in the liver, relying on the weight loss program, its purpose inside the frame, and its molecular make-up, the liver will either metabolize the nutrients or keep it.

Vitamin K is barely exceptional from its fats-soluble buddies. Rather than being saved or metabolized in the liver, diet plan K is the liver enzyme that makes it essential to liver feature.

Vitamin A deficiencies can result in rashes, ocular issues which incorporates night time blindness, and an impaired immune device. Vitamin D deficiencies can bring about an extended hazard of cardiovascular infection, rickets, bronchial bronchial asthma in children, cognitive impairment, and melancholy. Vitamin E deficiencies can motive muscle vulnerable factor, walking and coordination problems, immune system issues, and hassle with imaginative and prescient, together with numbness and tingling. Vitamin K deficiencies had been said to bring about excessive bleeding from cuts and wounds, smooth bruising, heavy menstrual intervals, oozing from the nose and gums, and blood inside the urine or stool.

This list of deficiency-associated health troubles is to outline clearly how essential nutrients are to the frame and commonplace fitness. If your liver is overtaxed or in some way damaged, storing and metabolizing vitamins can grow to be more difficult. Vitamin deficiencies aren't just due to now not eating diet plan-wealthy elements, dietary dietary supplements, or being out within the surroundings. They can also be the cease result of the body not being able to technique vitamins, which may stem from liver issues.

Drug Metabolism

A commonplace remedy for pretty some considered one of a kind signs and signs and ailments in modern-day treatment is the use of chemical tablets and pharmaceuticals. These pills have an important position on the subject of physical fitness. The liver moreover has an vital feature in how the ones medicinal pills and pills engage with the frame.

For the ones drug treatments and tablets to be powerful inside the frame, they want to undergo a metabolic method. This method permits to release their compounds into the body and lets in the frame to machine the compounds and then benefit the blessings from the drugs. Since tablets are commonly artificial with some chemical components, they're able to have small doses of poisonous debris that want to be filtered out of the body. If the ones particles aren't filtered out, they might building up and begin to reason extraordinary issues.

The liver performs a top position in not most effective metabolizing tablets and medicinal capsules but also in filtering out the waste and doubtlessly poisonous debris. Through a -section manner, the liver can spoil down and metabolize the medicinal tablets. The kidneys and gut are also beneficial in drug metabolism.

When it includes properly breaking down medicines and filtering out the waste, many elements make a contribution to right metabolic strategies. Age, gender, interactions amongst pills, being pregnant, diabetes, kidney infection, liver illness, genetics, and infection can also affect drug metabolism. In regards to liver health, some of these elements may be lessened or soothed via having a wholesome, sturdy liver.

Bilirubin Metabolism

Heme is a porphyrin elegance compound that consists of iron. It paperwork the non-protein part of hemoglobin and one-of-a-type natural molecules. Hemoglobin is a protein molecule in red blood cells. As a part of the red blood cells, hemoglobin is a completely essential protein molecule within the body. Heme is surely as vital, being part of the hemoglobin make-up.

The liver is one organ that performs a high position in the breakdown of heme. Other organs that play a role in hemolysis, the breakdown of heme, encompass the spleen and bone marrow. The hemolysis way breaks heme down into biliverdin, that is further damaged down into bilirubin. Once in the bilirubin form, it's miles secreted with the aid of the usage of bile through feces. Some bilirubin is reabsorbed via the use of manner of intestine bacteria or to be a part of enterohepatic waft.

This filtration manner is vital to the fitness of the blood and circulatory device. All cells within the frame undergo a technique of use, feature, and demise, which encompass blood cells. When a cellular reaches the stop of its lifestyles, it wants to be properly recycled or eliminated. The liver becomes that recycle-and-elimination catalyst for plenty types of cells inside the frame. This is the way it plays a function in blood purification.

Other Functions

Other important talents of the liver consist of the thyroid hormone feature and coping with the synthesis of plasma proteins and clotting factors of all intrinsic and extrinsic pathways, except element VIII.

The thyroid is an endocrine gland this is responsible for the manufacturing of some of hormones which can be critical to the body. These hormones effect the metabolism, inner frame temperature, and growth and development of the body. Having the liver assist regulate and manipulate thyroid hormone production is astronomically crucial to ordinary health and nicely-being.

Hopefully, you could now see how the liver plays its detail nearly about different crucial systems and methods in the body. It has a position in bodily talents which may be in definitely excellent cavities of the frame. An organ that has such strong relationships at some degree in the body have to be official and cared for.

A liver detox is considered one way to cleanse the liver and help to manual the organ simply so it may function at its maximum reliable degrees. However, there are way of life adjustments which may be beneficial to lengthy-time period liver fitness. That method that if you have have been given completed your liver detox or cleanse, you'll need to take measures for your life with weight loss plan, exercising, and different healthy modifications on the way to make sure your liver remains healthful long time.

As your liver strengthens through the years, you'll see massive enhancements in bodily fitness, and you can even see a few persistent or lengthy-term conditions starting to clear up.

How to Know If a Liver Detox Is Right for You

Before getting too deep into the concept of a liver detox, permit's go over what the time period "detox" method, what the intention of a detox is, and whilst and why you want to go through a detox software. Before we will talk about detoxes, we need to first speak about pollutants within the frame.

What are pollutants? "Toxin" is a specifically blanket term that covers the accumulation of any substance inside the body that could result in health troubles or undesirable thing effects. Most of the time, the body can flush pollution out on its personal. One of the components of these functions is the liver. Some of the commonplace pollution that human beings are exposed to every day encompass caffeine, alcohol, heavy metals, pollution, acids, bases, and medicinal tablets.

When the body is performing at excellent fitness, pollution don't have the hazard to build up or purpose problems. However, filtration and detox talents within the body can become impaired truly from each day existence. Exposure to positive forms of meals, environmental elements, capsules, and scientific troubles can bring about an impairment of body filtration structures. When the pollution begin to accumulate, the body has to artwork two times as hard to clear out them out.

If the buildup is a end result of some form of harm, collectively with a medical condition or extended-time period use of a remedy, then your frame may not be able to lure up with the toxin removal. Additionally, if the body has to paintings instances as hard to get rid of pollution and hold up with continued exposure, the organs in your body start to get overtaxed, like the liver. An overtaxed organ is heaps much less effective and might start to located on out or smash down. This is why the liver can also moreover have lasting damage from the overconsumption of alcohol. It can't preserve up with the filtration of pollutants from alcohol intake, which in the end pushes the liver into failure.

Just to be smooth, lots of the pollution that we're exposed to frequently are in innocent portions. Heavy metals like lead, mercury, and cadmium in addition to materials like arsenic are present in some of environmental strategies, such as in the pesticides which can be used commercially or in pollutants from factories. Cigarette smoke is a few different supply of these toxic substances, as is meals, in a few instances, in particular fine forms of fish which may be excessive in mercury ranges. In moderation and with the frame filtering pollution out well, those substances don't growth or motive problems.

Unfortunately, it is very smooth on this aspect in time to have the frame systems and organs conflict with their primary abilities. This is concerning the over-prescribing of drug treatments, smooth get proper of entry to to risky junk meals, the use of stronger and poisonous pesticides, and an boom in environmental pollutants. Overexposure to any of these substances can result in toxin buildup in the body. Some heavy metals, in more, can even inhibit the systems and methods which can be accountable for casting off them. This serves to exacerbate the hassle.

In a few times, heavy metals can compete with the natural absorption of minerals within the frame. This outcomes in toxic buildups and an ever-growing deficiency inside the minerals that your body desires.

It is sincere to mention that toxin buildup within the body is not top and might result in a number of fitness problems and worries. So, the question will become, how do you dispose of the pollution from your frame?

Simple, a detox.

The liver is considered the second one-hardest running organ inside the body, after the ever-pumping coronary coronary heart. So, at the equal time as you come back to the realization that it's time for a detox cleanse, you have to understand that the cause of a detox is to assist useful useful resource the organs in your body so that you can filter the pollution. With your liver, you need to offer sufficient help and treatment that the liver can do its manner with out being overtaxed but moreover hold up with right toxin filtration.

There are a number of supplemental detox plans out on the market these days. They market it a quick body flush and detox so that it will "reboot" your liver or specific organs and systems. These detox applications promote it a quick manner to lose weight, decrease ldl cholesterol, or restore the liver. While some of them can be effective, a actual body detox and cleanse is a more involved commitment that extends beyond a unmarried spherical of a supplemental detox.

A right detox software calls for a determination and willingness to change your manner of existence. You won't get at once outcomes, however the greater you decorate yourself and support your tool, the greater you could word the adjustments to your body. This trade can from time to time be diffused, however over time, it's miles difficult to deny the benefits and the effects.

You might not are privy to it, however your liver could be supplying you with signs and symptoms and signs that you need to pursue a detox software program software. A buildup of pollutants in your gadget can bring about mood adjustments, digestive issues, deteriorating organs, headaches, fatigue, infertility, reduced immune machine characteristic, troubles with mental clarity, and tingling in the direction of the body. Other problems can gift as uncommon bloating, rapid and unexplained weight advantage, trouble dropping weight inspite of healthy dietweight-reduction plan and exercising, modifications in complexion or pores and pores and pores and skin discoloration, heartburn, acid reflux sickness, digestive troubles, excessive perspiration, lack of inner homeostasis, and extraordinary lipid panels. These are all potential symptoms and symptoms and signs that your liver is suffering to smooth out pollutants from the body.

There are a few times in which you could need to don't forget a detox software even in case you haven't been experiencing any signs and symptoms and signs and symptoms. If you're having problem conceiving, are often uncovered to terrible satisfactory air, paintings with metals or chemical substances, have a residence that became constructed in advance than 1978, or live in a residence with vintage, previous plumbing, you then definately have to hold in mind a detox. These events can bring about toxin exposure, particularly heavy metals. If you have got troubles, you may even perform an at-home heavy metals blood test to peer if there may be a buildup of those toxic metals on your bloodstream.

It is surely simply well worth noting that heavy metals aren't the only forms of pollution that may growth to your body. If you've got got any of the above signs and symptoms or times in your existence, going through a liver detox software can assist. Not handiest does it help to lessen toxin buildup for your body, but it could furthermore help enhance your everyday health through manner of introducing more healthy behavior into your way of existence. This will save you toxin buildups inside the destiny and hold your organs functioning in a healthful way with out overtaxing them.

Chapter 2: Nine Signs Your Liver Is Unhappy

Oftentimes, whilst the frame is experiencing some type of ache, soreness, or sickness, it is only a symptom or sign of a few thing else taking place. These phrases—symptom and sign—are phrases which might be going to be used frequently in this ebook whilst discussing livers and possible dysfunctions. In the clinical undertaking, a symptom is an uncommon effect that is first-class felt or measurable from the angle of the character feeling it. A signal is a measurable impact or visible effect in the frame that may be observed via an outside supply, like a scientific expert.

For example, a headache could be considered a symptom due to the fact handiest the individual experiencing the headache is acquainted with the pain, soreness, or severity. A signal might be excessive blood pressure because of the fact that is a physical nation that can be measured and positioned by means of using the use of scientific tool and blood exams.

While the clinical region has advanced substantially over the last few hundred years, there have moreover been some setbacks. Medical experts who've a sturdy aspect, together with osteopaths, radiologists, or neurosurgeons, get immersed in their problem and now and again lose sight of the huge image. This way that a affected character may also have a list of signs that they track, and a consultant may not be capable of hyperlink them together if any of them effect body elements that don't coincide with their robust aspect.

Maybe you or someone has all over again to a scientific physician over and over with a listing of signs and symptoms and signs and symptoms that address continual ache, ache, digestion problems, or any variety of various problems. While those signs and symptoms and symptoms can be very telling approximately what is going on in the frame, the cutting-edge scientific vicinity frequently discredits symptoms and signs due to the fact they could't be measured. They look for signs and symptoms of illnesses or disorder, and if they'll't discover any, they write off the patient, which can be disturbing.

With the way the medical concern separates the body into such severa splendid additives (e.G. Pores and pores and skin, bones, joints, muscular tissues, organs, hormones, and neurons), it could be tough to take into account that all body additives are related and that organs just like the liver may be impacted through manner of manner of such loads of special bodily structures.

The scientific area is usually developing and evolving, and it's miles becoming clearer that there are flaws in the tool with the deviation amongst signs and symptoms and symptoms. A lot of people have encountered unsatisfactory reports with medical specialists in contemporary years, and loads of have decided to turn to extra holistic tactics. Holistic refers to an method that treats the complete man or woman or the entire body. This concept is what has paved the manner for extra statistics to pop out almost about liver detox plans and entire-frame cleanses for fitness and fitness.

Let's have a have a look at an instance of techniques a holistic method can be powerful. If a affected character goes to their medical doctor with issues about their thyroid, and the scientific medical doctor determines that the thyroid isn't generating hormones correctly, the affected man or woman will possibly be prescribed a medicinal drug to deal with the thyroid or to make artificial thyroid hormones. However, as we cited in Chapter 1, troubles with the liver can effect the thyroid and hormone manufacturing. The medicine can also help balance the thyroid, but if the hassle is in the liver, then it obtained't clear up the hassle, opposite it, or make it go away.

A holistic technique to thyroid troubles could be to don't forget the body as an entire and function a study what components of the frame can and do effect the thyroid reduce loose the gland itself. Then the entire body is dealt with with a focal point on those elements which is probably immediately related to the thyroid. So, at the same time as searching at a liver detox plan, it has a sturdy interest at the liver, but the strategies carried out, like diet and workout, also are focused at the fitness and nicely being of the whole body. This is what maintains the liver's functionality and keeps it healthy lengthy-term.

The variations between modern-day medicine and holistic remedy are what bring about the incorrect statistics about the frame. It is also why organs just like the liver aren't discussed in big care or annual physicals. Just to make clean, there are plenty of conditions in which "what you spot is what you get." That way that the signs and symptoms and signs and signs and signs and symptoms that have supplied themselves are at once related to the area they take area in. However, this isn't usually the case, particularly with regard to chronic and recurrent situations.

The different problem with symptoms and signs and symptoms and signs and symptoms and symptoms is that sometimes some of the same symptoms and signs and symptoms and signs and signs and symptoms and symptoms can gift themselves, however in exceptional human beings, they is probably related to sincerely particular troubles. This is each distinct drawback to modern remedy. Doctors frequently have a definitive idea of methods the frame abilities and what signs and symptoms or symptoms correlate to particular illnesses and illnesses. This method gets rid of the creativity this is required for making unusual diagnoses further to thinking of that all bodies are awesome and react and behave otherwise.

Since holistic medicinal drug and treatments approach the frame as a whole, they're much more likely to investigate every symptom and sign as a separate entity to locate the supply. This facilitates to prevent misdiagnosis if the symptoms and signs and symptoms and signs and signs and symptoms and signs and symptoms aren't what are generally seen for the ailment or trouble.

Misdiagnosis is, unluckily, common. Several years inside the past, a chum's daughter have become experiencing excessive knee ache. It modified into so awful she ought to rarely stand or walk. She needed to move on medical go away from her hobby and come to be spending most of her days sitting or mendacity down. In her teenagers, she'd had a bilateral knee state of affairs (each knees) with regard to her patella (kneecap). Her dad and mom took her back to the osteopath who had dealt with an appropriate knee situation.

The osteopath become a notable clinical medical doctor and a frontrunner in his challenge. However, without even analyzing this more younger female, he watched her stroll at some stage in the room and proclaimed that it wasn't the identical knee problem. So, he referred her to a rheumatologist thinking she had early-onset rheumatoid arthritis. Keep in mind that this journey commenced with this young woman going to her number one care scientific medical doctor, who referred her to the osteopath. It took over weeks to get an appointment. Now, she needed to wait each other and a half of of of weeks to get in with the rheumatologist.

After over a month of being shuffled spherical and referred, she ultimately were given her appointment. When the rheumatologist poked round at her kneecaps, he cautioned her that she didn't have arthritis, that 23-one year-olds don't get rheumatoid arthritis so all of sudden, and that she became tormented by the equal knee trouble that had plagued her in her kids. The state of affairs the osteopath so hopefully not noted.

This anecdote is an amazing example of the way specialists can overlook about signs and symptoms that don't correspond to what they expect to appearance. The osteopath come to be so happy that he have become seeing a special state of affairs based totally totally on the symptoms that had manifested, he didn't even do a physical exam on her knees. Fortunately, this more youthful female became capable of get right remedy for her knees, and she or he has lived consequences for over 5 years without any relapses.

Since the liver has connections to such some of organs, organ structures, and frame skills, the identical trouble can provide you with medical doctors if the liver is misbehaving or suffering. Modern treatment definitely has its location and its benefits, however one of the incredible methods you could help yourself is to take preventative measures in your entire frame, in particular for the organs that art work so tough for your frame, similar to the liver and coronary coronary heart.

Signs and Symptoms That Might Indicate Your Liver Is Struggling

As formerly stated, there aren't any lessen-and-dried signs or signs that truly advocate a trouble with the liver. Short of a liver disease evaluation, it can be difficult to

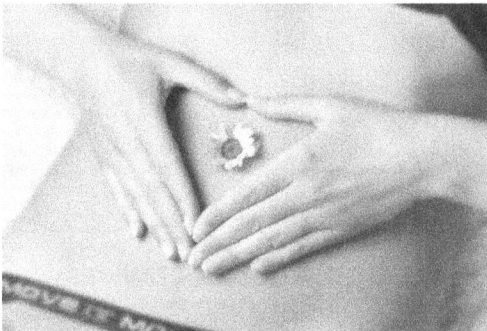

pinpoint the reason of your symptoms and signs and symptoms and symptoms and signs and symptoms. That being stated, there are a few not unusual symptoms and signs that the liver is struggling. This won't be the identical for anybody, however on common, these are the 9 essential symptoms and signs and symptoms that have been found and said.

Let's check what may also moreover imply the liver is overtaxed and in need of a detox:

•Unexpected or rapid weight benefit or an incapacity to shed pounds with weight loss plan and exercising

•Unusual belly bloating (no longer associated with other symptoms much like the menstrual cycle)

•Heartburn

•Poor sleep

•Mysterious starvation or cravings

•Overheating of the body or a loss of inner homeostasis

•Changes in complexion or pores and pores and skin discoloration

•Sluggish liver

•Chemical sensitivities or hypersensitive reactions

Since an organ similar to the liver is so critical to the body and physical capabilities, at the same time as it begins to warfare, symptoms and signs and signs and signs and symptoms received't be scarce. Toxins take some time to accumulate inside the body, and over the years, specific symptoms and symptoms and symptoms and signs and symptoms and signs and symptoms take vicinity. It must begin with clean heartburn or digestive pain. People regularly overlook approximately those less concerned or a bargain lots less hindering signs and signs and learn how to live with them.

Unfortunately, even small signs and symptoms are the body trying to inform you that a few component isn't pretty right. Does this endorse you need to go to the scientific physician every time you have a case of heartburn? Unless you have an already diagnosed clinical state of affairs that results in heartburn and is probably life-threatening, this isn't recommended. However, you want to take a step lower back and reflect onconsideration on what might be causing it. Maybe you're ingesting substances which can be excessive in acids, like tomatoes and warm peppers. If you may reduce again on the consumption of those excessive acid substances, your heartburn might in all likelihood show drastic improvement.

So, symptoms and signs and symptoms and signs and symptoms and signs are your frame's way of communicating that some component isn't quite right. If you are presently experiencing or have experienced any of the nine signs or signs stated inside the above listing, there may be a threat that your liver wants to be cleansed and detoxed. An sad liver only receives unhappier. A not unusual misconception is that if a sign or symptom is neglected and goes away, then the hassle is resolved. This is unfaithful. Usually, all which means that is that the body has decided a way to capture up on the ache or soreness.

Massage therapists see this all the time. A purchaser might also come to them for chronic foot pain. After numerous classes, they will discover the deliver of the pain is an vintage surgical scar on the once more. Over the years, the client unconsciously adjusted how they walked and sat to seize up on the ache from the surgical scar. Eventually, the pain traveled from the again, down the legs, and into the toes wherein it settled and feature come to be persistent.

The equal element can appear with organs. If you're running on figuring out wherein your signs and symptoms and signs and signs and symptoms originate from, an top notch location to start is to song them. You can use a pocket book, cell telephone app, or laptop software to make a list of symptoms and signs and signs and symptoms. Then music on the same time as you be conscious them, how lengthy they final, and the without delay stimulus that angry them (if you can determine the purpose). Over time, you may see styles that emerge, which let you get inside the route of the premise reason, along with an overtaxed liver.

Another choice to hold in thoughts is to partake in a liver cleanse software application if any of the above signs and symptoms or symptoms and symptoms and symptoms have made themselves recognized in your life. A liver detox weight loss plan isn't going to be risky on your frame if your liver doesn't need the extra assist. It can simplest assist. Now, making those modifications for your lifestyles can result in a lack of unfastened time and propose more art work and attempt. You might not be willing to take that bounce without greater concrete evidence that your liver is in need of a few assist.

That is also a legitimate function to take. If you aren't satisfied, attempt tracking a number of the symptoms and symptoms and symptoms earlier than leaping proper proper right into a liver detox plan. At the forestall of this financial ruin, trying out your liver may also be mentioned as a further technique for identifying if a liver detox plan is right for you. Please additionally hold in thoughts that the signs and signs and symptoms and symptoms and signs and symptoms and symptoms above are only a handful of issues that can upward push up from an overtaxed liver.

The Connection Between Liver Disease and Mental Health, Depression, and Anxiety

Going once more to the distinction amongst symptoms and signs and signs and signs and signs, there is one clinical problem that is nearly surely primarily based mostly on signs and symptoms and signs and signs and symptoms and signs and symptoms felt and recommended thru sufferers. This scientific area is likewise considered one of the most taboo fields. While interest is developing round it, standards like highbrow health, depression, and tension are nonetheless labeled with a wonderful deal of stigma, ridicule, and skepticism.

Mental fitness is difficult to song and trace as it varies so extensively from individual to man or woman and facilities almost totally on invisible signs and symptoms and symptoms. There are nonetheless those in modern society who say "it is all of their head" or who are otherwise convinced highbrow fitness is an excuse or a made-up purpose for human beings to behave a sure manner to justify how they revel in.

It is unlucky that there may be such controversy spherical intellectual health because of the truth there are various conditions that have arisen out of the intellectual health field which have confirmed that the thoughts can effect the physical body, belief patterns, and behaviors. The thoughts works off of chemical secretions and electric powered impulses. If the ones impulses and secretions are in any way impaired or imbalanced, then the mind can emerge as awful within the same manner the body can end up risky if the liver isn't working well.

Liver infection and its connection to intellectual health, despair, and anxiety has been cited at some point of numerous medical and psychological corporations. It has been placed that those who have liver disease are more susceptible to tension, depression, and special highbrow fitness conditions.

In reality, throughout younger populations, it has been determined that teenagers with liver disease or chronic liver issues show a far higher rate of melancholy and tension or stress. A have a check finished in 2016 at a liver transplant health facility in London confirmed that the not unusual stressors protected troubles drowsing, lethargy, issues approximately cash, problems at school or artwork, anxiety, and coffee shallowness (Samyn, 2020, para 8).

It is usually advocated that younger age groups who are gift technique remedy for liver ailment or who have been thru a liver transplant take delivery of a further holistic treatment that doesn't really cope with the body however additionally allows to treat and heal the thoughts to prevent a rise in intellectual health situations due to persistent liver illness.

While this take a look at end up based totally totally on young adults who have been already diagnosed with liver illness, there may be moreover proof to suggest that psychosocial stress performs a position in inflicting liver sickness, extra in particular persistent viral hepatitis. Hepatitis is a liver-attacking situation. It has lengthy been positioned that everyone being treated for chronic infection that consequences in a traumatic existence or emotional kingdom or who evaluations publicity to plenty of stressors shows a dramatic decline in bodily health. This concept that pressure may be risky to the immune tool or perhaps wreck down the frame isn't truly novel.

However, research finished more presently on animals and people have confirmed smooth, definitive hyperlinks among pressure and the way it could make contributions to the development of viral hepatitis. These equal studies went on to expose that strain also can get worse the inflammatory nature of liver cirrhosis. Since the liver plays a feature within the immune tool and numerous of the inter- and intra-mobile mechanisms, stress to the frame and feelings can motive a more rapid development of liver pathologies (Vere et al., 2009).

You can see in reality how the liver can be impacted by way of the use of stress and anxiety that is regularly perceived as "normal" in nowadays's society. You can also see how, at the turn facet, issues in the liver can make contributions to the manifestation of intellectual health issues, like depression. So, the way you cope with your body and stay your lifestyles may additionally need to have an immediate impact on your liver, resulting in liver sickness. Also, mild intellectual health situations can be a signal or symptom that your liver is beginning to war and no longer capable of hold up collectively along with your way of existence.

Speaking from a holistic approach, the whole lot in the frame is established. Whether it is through connective tissue, the apprehensive device, or blood go together with the go with the flow, the frame is all linked. Even anxiety, depression, and responses to pressure are your body's manner of saying some thing isn't quite proper. In a society in which we are nearly recommended to stress ourselves out on a every day foundation running grueling jobs, preserving up with own family and community, balancing chores with pals, seeking to squeeze in some personal time, and paying bills on time, pressure becomes a major fitness element for the body.

Some of what you are going to discover at the same time as studying about the liver detox and weight loss plan software is the manner to control pressure to help save you it from turning into a trouble on your liver. Additionally, when you have struggled with depression and tension at some stage in your life, you could need to function that in your symptom or sign list of motives you want to pursue a liver detox software.

Test Your Liver

If you want definitive evidence earlier than identifying to embark on a manner of lifestyles exchange that becomes your long-time period liver detox and fitness plan, then you can consider having your liver tested for issues.

There are some at-domestic blood checks you can take to test at the reputation of your liver. Some, like Thorne's Heavy Metal At-Home Blood Test, may show a presence of heavy metals within the blood.

Various tests diploma a desire of factors, which encompass degrees of:

•Alanine transaminase (ALT)

•Aspartate aminotransferase (AST)

•Alkaline phosphatase (ALP)

•Albumin

•Bilirubin

When you go to the health practitioner, you could need a greater complete examination precise to the liver to decide if whatever is incorrect. This may also want to embody a natural examination, ultrasound of the liver, or a hepatic biopsy. While the ones tests and exam procedures will be inclined to be in regards to excessive symptoms and signs and symptoms, you can discover at-domestic blood check kits with a purpose to show show for the indexed gadgets above.

If you do have essential problems about your liver, strive an at-domestic blood check. You ought to likely need to are searching for advice from an authorized scientific professional relying on the effects. Or, you can decide that it is time so you should make the determination to a liver detox diet regime.

Chapter 3: Introduction To The Liver Detox Program

If you've been looking around for records about a liver detox, you've in all likelihood encountered a whole lot of distinct facts approximately the professionals and cons of detoxification, some medical data that would seem contradictory, and severa precise paths you can take to attain your detox dreams.

Like in maximum situations, there are a whole lot of different approaches to move approximately meeting your goals. A lot of the liver detox and cleanse packages spherical, specifically those that include dietary supplements and strict fasting or "deep cleaning" strategies, are intended for a brief-time period liver flush and reboot. The liver detox plan that changed into designed and built for this ebook is for lengthy-term liver health. It does begin with a brief-time period deep cleanse, but the conventional goal is to provide a way of life converting plan a good way to manual your liver for many years to return once more.

Just to make clean, the supplement detoxes and their short-flush strategies might be powerful for a few human beings and can be the overall intention. In the fast time period, they may be quite useful. However, "flushing" the frame of pollution over 3 days or one week doesn't alternate the quantity of pollution which can be moving into your frame on a each day basis because of your lifestyle and what you're uncovered to environmentally.

Short-time period liver flushes can grow to be complicated for the frame if used constantly as a way to lower toxin buildup. Between the fasting and honestly particular nutritional necessities, they aren't designed to manipulate toxin buildup in the body. A short-term detox or cleanse is designed to rid your body of amassed pollutants so you can start with a easy slate. Once the slate is easy, no matter the reality that, if you pass lower lower back to the identical behavior as earlier than, it turns into gunked up with pollution once more.

This is what devices this liver detox software program apart.

This liver detox and cleansing software program software is supposed to flush pollution out of your system and additionally manage the big shape of toxins which is probably positioned into your frame frequently. Since there are so many one among a kind resources of pollution, like air pollution, horrible eating water, and lead paint in an vintage house, you gained't be capable of control each single toxic element that you are exposed to, however you don't need to.

A lengthy-time period liver useful resource software starts with a short flush however then moreover offers records, facts, and step-with the resource of-step commands on way of existence modifications that can help you restrict your toxin consumption and because of this shield your body from toxin buildups. This liver detox software takes it one step in addition through bringing inside the holistic approach of helping the frame, mind, and emotions while you are cleaning and striving for a greater wholesome destiny.

What Is a Liver Detox?

A liver detox is in fact a way to flush pollutants out of your body, especially the liver. It's commonly no longer a complicated technique, even though it does require try to your detail. Hopefully, after reading the primary chapters, you recognize the signs and signs and symptoms and signs and signs and signs and symptoms that would allude to wanting a liver cleanse. If you're even though analyzing, you've in all likelihood determined a liver cleanse is right for you, but you will be wondering why this software and what the unique blessings are. Some of the benefits of liver detoxes have been touched on before, however under is a whole listing of the advantages to a liver detox software program and lengthy-time period liver beneficial resource.

A liver detox:

•Naturally boosts strength (no greater counting on caffeine!)

•Removes luggage and dark circles from underneath the eyes and decreases the redness and puffiness across the eyes

•Clears pores and pores and skin (this is going for zits, blotches, eczema, touch dermatitis, and precise skin conditions which may be perceived as topical)

•Normalizes the metabolism (which incorporates food processing, nutrient extraction, and bowel actions)

•Normalizes body weight to a wholesome degree

•Brings blood levels of cholesterol to a wholesome area

•Removes tongue coating, improving the feel of flavor

•Helps guide the immune tool so it is able to higher preserve your body healthy and secure from pathogens, infections, viruses, and micro organism

•Reduces swellings and edemas (fluid buildups) inside the body

•Keeps the body from bruising effects

These blessings, in turn, produce other affects at the frame. For instance, regulating metabolism, digestion, and body weight may be an essential part of dealing with kind 2 diabetes. While kind 2 diabetes may also additionally constantly require insulin use, coping with body weight, metabolism, and digestion can lessen the quantity of insulin that is required daily, furthermore saving coins in the long run.

If you've got chronic pores and pores and skin conditions that don't appear to have a "root" reason, then it is able to be due to toxin buildups within the body. Acne is an increasingly commonplace topical pores and pores and skin problem in which the supply is regularly unknown. Teenagers and adults can struggle with pimples. No depend how masses you wash your face, take acne medicinal drug, or lessen your sugar consumption, you could no matter the fact that war, and the liver might be the culprit. If the liver isn't nicely clearing the body of pollution, they occur in other strategies, which include acne, eczema, and other pores and skin conditions. Despite the epidermis being at the outdoor of the frame, if the indoors of the body isn't functioning nicely, then the outdoor will display symptoms and signs and symptoms.

Many people battle with weight loss. They undergo cycles of diets and workout and grow to be no longer making any progress.

Sometimes, it isn't approximately focused on weight loss mainly. Just like with the pores and skin conditions, the disability to shed pounds can be a byproduct of an sad liver.

When it includes a healthy immune gadget, the place is whole of pathogens. They come as viruses, micro organism, infections, and ailments. The frame's very own protection machine in opposition to those distant places invaders which can be looking for to harm it's miles the immune tool. With a wholesome immune device, your frame can be masses higher at fighting off the ones pathogens. Even in case you get exposed, you could stand a better threat of now not growing signs and symptoms and symptoms or having intense reactions because of the truth your body is capable of keep the pathogens from inflicting harm.

That being said, there are diagnosed pathogens which are extensively sturdy or new, and the frame doesn't understand them as risky and can't combat them off. A healthful immune machine doesn't recommend you aren't prone to getting unwell; it surely approach you could now not get sick as frequently or the signs and symptoms and symptoms won't be as immoderate.

There are many benefits to a liver detox plan. The provided list is definitely an creation to what a liver detox can do for you.

A Word of Warning

A phrase of caution in advance than you soar into the number one liver cleanse you phrase.

It isn't always unusual in recent times to go into the health section of a grocery keep, complement keep, or all-herbal marketplace and see classified ads for entire detox packages. You should purchase a detox container costing $50 or more that consists of severa dietary dietary supplements and commands on how to complete the detox software program. These bins are usually only prepared with enough dietary supplements to closing for a few days to each week, giving the effect that once the nutritional nutritional supplements are lengthy beyond, the detox is whole.

Unfortunately, a real cleanse that permits you to significantly gain the frame is a protracted-term willpower. Fixing years' well well really worth of stress and harm to the liver can't be resolved in only some days. So, be cautious of detox plans and programs that advertise "whole health" or "whole detox" in only a few days. Sometimes, those cleaning programs will bypass as an extended way as to say which you'll see a drastic distinction to your weight, clarity of pores and skin, and distinct common troubles. Those are very attractive advertising and marketing strategies, but with out proper study-up, they aren't going to appear.

The specific drawback to a liver detox in a container is that a few agencies use portions of dietary dietary supplements that can be risky to the frame or certainly one of a type organs or systems within the body. Some packages call for ingesting large quantities of juices. This can be volatile to sincerely anyone with diabetes or kidney disorder. Fasting is often part of the detox-in-a-container plan. If finished incorrectly, fasting can lead to weakness and fainting. Additionally, when you have liver damage from hepatitis B, fasting should make the harm worse. Even in spite of the fact that the supplemental detox in a topic idea is all-herbal and doesn't include prescribed drugs or heavy tablets, they're running from the mentality of right away gratification and on the spot fixes.

A liver detox is greater than a three- to seven-day cleansing software. It is extra than certainly detox nutritional nutritional dietary supplements and liquids. It isn't a one-time software program application that fixes the whole thing. This can be hard to surely be given once in a while due to the truth, in the age of generation and western remedy, immediately gratification is the favored very last outcomes whilst a person attempts some aspect new or wants to see a exchange. True change comes from exercise and dedication, despite the fact that. A real liver detox software is a lifestyle exchange with the choice to be healthful and help your liver characteristic.

What Is Our Liver Detox Program?

Our liver detox software program is going to begin you off with a seven-day liver flush. The flush is frequently going to be based totally completely mostly on healthy eating plan and fasting; but, it is also going to cover a few meditation strategies to help you preserve your highbrow and emotional health at the same time as your frame is detoxing. You also can acquire some easy workout plans which can be designed to beautify your metabolism and natural power. They received't be too intense or rigorous as your body is probably going to sense susceptible from the periods of fasting.

These seven days are going to be your first step towards liver fitness. The essential goal of this flush is largely to offer your liver a damage. It is designed to easy your body of pollutants brief after which extensively limit the range of pollution entering your body at that factor so your liver can relaxation and reboot. When your computer is a bit gradual, tech help continuously recommends rebooting the laptop as a primary step. It is how your computer unloads all of the "junk" documents or pointless buildup of records that is dragging down the internal processing. In terms of your liver, the primary seven-day flush is meant to do really that!

After the seven-day liver flush, you may have three days of meal plans, exercising, and meditation practices an excellent manner to attention on constructing your liver's health and assisting to restore any harm achieved to your liver before bringing it decrease again to complete function. These 3 days will basically be targeted on 3 food a day, with a few snacks, which might be completely designed for liver health.

So, after your liver is rebooted and your body is free of pollution, you need your liver to ease lower lower back into what desires to be carried out. Consider this like rehab or restoration for your liver. If you've ever broken a bone in an arm or leg or had critical surgical treatment, then you definitely simply truely understand that inside the convalescing approach, there is an element of physical treatment or rehab. Your frame essentially wants to be reminded a way to use that limb or body detail as soon because the lengthy restoration length is over. If your liver has been struggling for some time, you'll need to remind it what it looks as if to characteristic commonly. In doing so, you pork up and put together it to come back once more decrease lower back to full use, the same as you can a recovered damaged leg. Fortunately, for the reason that liver is an organ that doesn't require aware attempt to make it characteristic, 3 days of rehab have to be hundreds to get it once more into the swing of normality.

Once your three days of rejuvenation have ended, you will be given lengthy-time period instructions for keeping liver health. These lengthy-term plans will cowl your food plan with counseled normal food and snacks. It can also additionally cowl right exercise plans and techniques for keeping your self healthful and retaining your weight desires. You'll moreover accept greater meditation practices which can be going to retain to foster a wholesome and satisfactory attitude closer to your way of lifestyles modifications and your private health.

The prolonged-time period element of keeping liver health is meant to be a lifelong practice. Keeping your liver healthful indefinitely is going to behave as a excellent preventative in later existence. With age, the frame glaringly turns into extra vulnerable to fitness conditions. If your liver is stored strong and healthy, your frame can be plenty a whole lot much less at risk of age-related breakdowns of the immune system and different organ functions. It isn't always an answer for developing older, only a solution for long-term fitness and well-being.

There might be a phase of the detox plan that covers meals on your whole own family in case you're looking to keep anybody in your circle of relatives healthy as well. The step-with the useful resource of-step commands furnished also can even encompass useful facts about why those steps and techniques are implemented with reference to liver flushing, cleansing, and prolonged-term liver fitness.

During the seven-day flush, there may be pointers for liver-supporting dietary supplements that may be taken. The dietary supplements which can be recommended are going to be consistent, and they will embody any precautions to do not forget earlier than taking them. They aren't essential to our liver detox software program program; but, they will be able to assist facilitate the technique and assist your liver rebound a chunk quicker.

It is important to make the distinction amongst the ones advocated nutritional nutritional dietary dietary supplements and the liver detox in a area. Individual dietary dietary supplements, like milk thistle, are a pure supply of that herb. The equal is real of nutritional dietary supplements like omega-3s and minerals like zinc. They aren't a mixture or aggregate. They are capsuled out with wholesome proportions and feature commands for proper each day utilization. They also are truly non-compulsory in your use.

Before you get started out out together along with your liver detox software program application, it's far encouraged that you get a pocket e-book or mag to commit in your plan. If it's far much less complicated to preserve an virtual document of what you do and revel in, find out a suitable phone app or computer software program application that allows you to assist you to song your progress.

Not best can you operate this magazine to preserve notes on what you are supposed to be doing at which level of the detox plan you are in, but you may also use it to song adjustments in your frame. Recording particular emotions, sensations, and a few element you examine is a remarkable manner to song the subtle adjustments that might circulate overlooked. It can be very motivating to have notes in black and white that validate and verify your development.

This pocket e book serves a dual purpose, even though. If a few components of the program don't be just right for you or some paintings very well, you'll word and be able to alter your plan therefore. You'll be able to regularly section out subjects that don't benefit you and replace them with topics that do. Everyone's frame is particular, and additionally you can not have the identical fulfillment with pleasant techniques. That's flawlessly okay. Additionally, when you have any precise allergic reactions or preexisting conditions, you can want to shift and alter the plan in order that it stays wholesome for you.

You can maintain track of greater than in reality what occurs to your body bodily. You can also write down the thoughts and emotions you have were given in the course of the detox software. When your body starts offevolved offevolved to detox, you'll probable revel in mood swings or adjustments in mood. Writing approximately them assist you to to control them further to reflect on what you felt as you moved thru this gadget. Since there may be a meditation factor to this detox software, writing about thoughts, emotions, and studies from the meditations will decorate the holistic aspect of this gadget.

Notebooks and journals, in particular if they may be virtual, are with out difficulty transportable. That method you can maintain them with you although you can't preserve this e book with you. If you hold music of your doorstep-through-step plan to your pocket ebook, there aren't any excuses for not following the plan.

Check With Your Doctor Before Starting a Cleanse

Prior to committing to or beginning our liver detox program, you want to take a look at in together together together with your primary doctor or health care professional. If you have any preexisting conditions, that is vitally crucial. There are a few conditions which could't manage a liver detox, in particular when there is a fasting or juice/smoothie difficulty, as our software program consists of.

People with kidney ailment and diabetes should honestly address the juice consumption of a liver detox software cautiously and high-quality with the consent and moderation of a clinical health practitioner. If you've got any kidney sickness or acknowledged harm, preserve with warning and only with the express permission of a qualified healthcare organisation. Some kidney illnesses and harm may be aggravated thru the detox software steps.

It is vital to recognize what a liver detox and prolonged-term health plan can do for you, but while you don't forget that extended-time period fitness is the general purpose, you want to do it proper. If you're liable to food allergies, be cautious with the recipes in the occasion that they encompass components you haven't eaten earlier than. You may want to likely want to make substitutions to the recipes, however make certain to use complementary materials that gained't disrupt the cleanse or detox application.

Anyone with low blood strain, low iron, or a data of fainting ought to be cautious of the fasting portions and are seeking advice from a systematic physician or health care expert to make sure fasting is secure for them. Additionally, in case you're pregnant, in your health and your toddler's fitness, you will possibly remember preserving off on the detox utility until after your toddler is born, besides your health practitioner gives you the skip-in advance.

A preexisting condition doesn't routinely exclude you from being able to perform or gain from our liver detox utility. You want to make certain that it is going to advantage you in spite of the reality that, and that is why each person, even a person with out a preexisting circumstance, have to double-take a look at with their doctor earlier than starting. Your health is the general purpose, so make sure you stand to gain advantages earlier than starting.

Once you've carried out that, it's time to get began.

Chapter 4: A Liver Detox Program That Will Leave You Feeling Energized And Healthy

Welcome to the first steps of your liver detox software program software. To start, you'll begin with a distinctly intensive liver flush a good way to span seven days. For a whole week, you'll want to paste to this step-via using-step software to ensure that your frame is flushed of pollutants and your liver is prepared to refresh and work in the path of creating you greater healthful.

You'll notice that the seven-day flush is damaged down thru day. Each day is going to cover an outline of what you need to be doing on your flush on those days. This utility isn't supposed to disrupt your every day life. You might also additionally want to make some timing adjustments to work inside the meditations and the workout quantities. However, trendy, you won't want to put your life on hold or change your each day time desk.

Like the seven-day flush, the three-day rejuvenation plan has also been damaged down into precise days with easy commands at the way to address your liver on those days. The three days are a bit extra traumatic when it comes to genuine food because it's miles based on a plan that changed into advanced by way of a cirrhosis patient. You should possibly want to double-check your kitchen to ensure you have got the critical device or alternative gadget for the food coaching that includes this liver manual plan.

Even if you don't have masses of enjoy cooking, it's miles encouraged which you begin your very very own meal prep or ask for the assist of someone in your private home or a chum or member of the family who can put together dinner to assist train you. Part of the liver detox plan is to screen what goes into your frame. Purchasing premade factors or ordering takeout from eating places isn't going to have the same food fantastic, no matter the truth that the menu item appears or sounds identical to what you want to be making prepared.

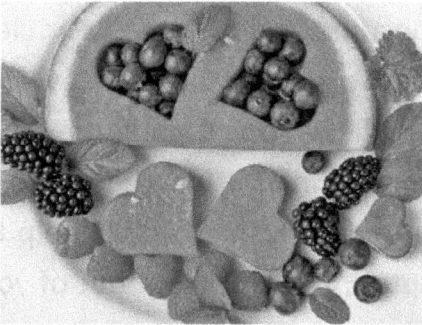

Please remember that at the identical time as you are detoxing, your body can also go through quite a few adjustments. Your moods is probably a touch greater complex or tumultuous. Overall, through the stop of the sizeable detox, you have to experience more energized, more wholesome, and more nice.

Seven-Day Liver Flush

To make certain that your liver flush is powerful, there are a few dos and don'ts to cowl so you are definitely organized for the technique. First and number one, you'll need to test the statistics approximately what to eat and drink. Then, inventory up your kitchen with the chocolates that you could consume and drink to your cleanse. If it is an desire, you would likely even need to get rid of the ones gadgets you may't devour and drink within the route of your week-extended flush. This will help to avoid the temptation to interrupt out of your flush food regimen.

Important "don'ts" in your seven-day flush encompass:

•Don't devour wheat and gluten. They are each gut irritants. Give your digestive device each week-long wreck.

•Don't devour milk and dairy. Milk is a not unusual food allergen, and the frame creates antibodies for it, stimulating and overtaxing your immune device. Milk additionally turns on the body to create extra mucus. After in step with week without dairy, you may probable even find that you're feeling so pinnacle you don't want to reintroduce it.

•Don't eat caffeine. As difficult as it is not to have your morning coffee or that afternoon cup of black tea, try to avoid it because of the reality caffeine is contributing on your liver's overtaxation. Caffeine is an addictive toxin that the liver works tough to flush out. Use this as an possibility to kick the addiction and repair your liver. Tip: If you actually cannot reduce caffeine from your each day life, keep on and not using a extra than cups of inexperienced tea a day. Green tea is complete of antioxidants, that are essential at some point of a cleanse, and isn't excellent excessive in caffeine content fabric. It is a notable line, so best walk it if there are no extraordinary alternatives.

•Don't drink alcohol. This is massive with regards to liver cleansing and liver health. Alcohol is arguably your liver's best enemy.

Cut it out for constant with week to clearly allow your liver rest.

•Don't devour processed sugars and processed meals. When possible, avoid food with sugars and sweeteners that aren't natural. Raw honey and pure maple syrup are unprocessed, herbal sugars. You can alternative them for exceptional sugars in case you'd like. Consuming loads of sugary food and processed factors heavy in preservatives can counteract what you are trying to do as sugar toilets down your strength tiers and processed components are plenty tougher to digest, contributing to more weight.

•Don't smoke cigarettes or vape. The chemicals in cigarette smoke and vaping juice intrude with the detox software program software. Plus, they may be bad for you and could reason different prolonged-term troubles.

•Don't consume quite a few saturated fat. Saturated fats and barbecued meat also are inhibitors to the liver flush method. Be conscientious of the amount of saturated fats you're consuming, and live far from the charcoal grill at some stage in your detox.

A few "dos" or conduct to choose up at the same time as you're operating on your seven-day liver flush encompass:

•Drink water constantly throughout the day. It will help keep wastes and fluids transferring through your system and get them removed out of your body. Staying hydrated may even help to facilitate the method. Tip: Drinking greater water necessarily results in extra toilet breaks. Plan due to this each time feasible.

•Eat superfoods. These might be included in greater detail .

Fruits which you'll need to eat loads of within the path of your detox encompass glowing apricots, cantaloupe, kiwi, peaches, papaya, citrus fruits, melons, pink grapes, mangoes, and berries of a huge range. Vegetables a great way to advantage your detox plan encompass peppers, beets, broccoli, artichokes, purple cabbage, Brussels sprouts, cauliflower, carrots, kale, pumpkin, cucumber, spinach, sweet potatoes, watercress, tomato, and bean and seed sprouts.

These are the superfoods. All of the above meals are immoderate in antioxidants, nutrients, protein, minerals, wholesome starches, wholesome fats, and materials like chlorophyll that permits to leech heavy metals and pollution from the body.

There are different components that you can eat at some point of a detox software program program, but they want to be fed on carefully. Limit your grain intake, and stick with complete grains which might be gluten-unfastened (e.G. Brown rice, quinoa, and oats). Limit your fish consumption to no extra than as soon as every day. Stick to fish like salmon, mackerel, anchovies, and sardines which can be appeared to be lower in mercury than distinct famous fish which include tuna and swordfish.

During the seven days of cleansing, you may have one serving each one-of-a-kind day of ingredients like bananas and potatoes. They have starches and chemical substances that imitate hormones like estrogen. These forms of materials want to be fed on with care inside the direction of a detox.

Nuts and seeds have to be fed on each day however in a single amount of approximately one handful. They are wealthy in natural, first rate fat and proteins. Nuts and seeds to devour embody Brazil nuts, almonds, pecans, hazelnuts, sunflower seeds, pumpkin seeds, flaxseed, chia seeds, and sesame seeds. You'll want to bear in thoughts switching to extra virgin olive oil as a cooking oil and using flaxseed oil or a few one of a kind cold-pressed seed oil for bloodless oil bases (like salad dressings).

There are meals to truely keep away from in some unspecified time in the future of your liver detox flush as well. As said above, avoid all milk and dairy, together with cheese, yogurt, ice cream, and cream. You should moreover avoid meat in the course of those seven days. Red meat, hen and bird, red meat, eggs—take a spoil from all meat for seven days. Grains like rye, wheat, spelt, and barley all have gluten in them, so keep away from those grains as properly.

Additionally, you shouldn't be eating salt at some point of this seven-day flush. Avoid ingredients that have sodium. Stay far from hydrogenated fats, preservatives, synthetic sweeteners, and processed sugars, further to fried meals, spices, and dried fruits.

It seems like lots to preserve tune of, but the seven-day breakdown beneath gives you the steps to make use of this statistics in a wholesome way.

Optional: Supplements that you could take in the course of your seven-day cleanse encompass a multivitamin and a entire antioxidant supplement. The superfoods and the healthy eating plan recommendations on your seven-day plan all encompass excessive stages of nutrients, minerals, and antioxidants. It isn't important to take them, but they are able to give your flush and liver an introduced enhance.

Antioxidants combat the frame's internal and outside publicity to oxidants. Oxidants, in abundance, can motive cell damage, triggering many conditions together with inflammation or perhaps most cancers. Regardless of whether or not or now not or now not you're doing a liver cleanse, antioxidants are important to health and properly being. However, a proper, balanced weight-reduction plan gets you the ones vitamins and antioxidants with out the resource of nutritional supplements.

Some specific non-obligatory liver-helping dietary supplements consist of milk thistle extract, dandelion extract, glutamine, and MSM. Milk thistle extract binds to pollutants to help get rid of them from the frame and could increase glutathione to preserve pollutants moving via the frame until they're eliminated.

MSM is a sulfur compound. It is a liver-helping compound that also aids in the production of glutathione. Dandelion extract has been used for hundreds of years in severa natural remedies and through herbalists. While it's miles typically taken into consideration a weed, it is also a very beneficial plant. Dandelion extract allows the liver and moreover allows with the manufacturing of bile. Bile, as mentioned in Chapter 1, plays a outstanding position in liver characteristic and detoxifying the body.

If making a decision to take any nutrients and supplements, double- and triple-check the dosage and utilization instructions at the bottle. Also, look for any capability contraindications and conflicts with preexisting situations. If you don't see any apparent notes but have a preexisting scenario, seek advice from your health practitioner or primary care clinical doctor to decide the safety of taking the ones supplements. Be privy to the reality that our liver program doesn't require the use of any vitamins or nutritional dietary supplements to paintings.

When a cleanse refers to "fasting," it doesn't imply to avoid meals for prolonged periods. This sort of fasting is as regards to lowering out processed and terrible components and sticking to raw, healthful substances such as slight end end result and greens, as defined above. Quantities of meals are contracted down as nicely.

In the breakdown of every day, there might be particular recipes referenced. The real recipes, on the aspect of others that aren't referenced especially, that can be included in your liver flush and rejuvenation plans might be protected in the bonus financial disaster of this ebook. The advantages of every superfood might be blanketed in parentheses, so experience free to pick out out the handiest that fits your desires top notch.

Meditations may also be stated, and the instructions for those meditations can also be covered within the "recipes" bonus financial disaster. Use the notes in that economic destroy to examine along and perform the meditation nicely.

A useful tip for starting your seven-day flush is to start on a weekend day, like a Saturday, so that you can exercising getting within the swing without procedure expectations. This gives you some time to regulate to this new plan.

00005.Jpeg

Day 1

Start your day off with one of the following cleaning, detoxifying beverages:

•Cucumber-mint detox

•Orange, carrot, and ginger detox

Follow up your detox beverage with a small bowl of mixed glowing berries. Any combination will do:

•Blueberries

•Strawberries

•Raspberries

•Gooseberries

•Goji berries

•Blackberries

•Acai berries

•Cranberries

•Grapes

For lunch, enjoy a heat cup of dandelion tea with raw honey (liver and bile assist, a herbal sweetener that allows with seasonal allergic reactions).

Have yourself a handful of nuts and seeds (high in protein, healthful fat, wholesome oils, and antioxidants). Mix any of the subsequent nuts and seeds:

•Pecans

•Hazelnuts

•Brazil nuts

•Almonds

•Pumpkin seeds

•Sunflower seeds

•Chia seeds

•Flaxseeds

•Sesame seeds

Also, eat a smooth apricot and carrot sticks along with your nuts and seeds (antioxidants, detoxing, and wholesome) and a detoxifying "drink your vegetables" fruit and vegetable juice (full of nutrients K and other important nutrients).

Take a 5-minute walk out of doors (weather permitting). If you may't stroll outside and there's no to be had indoor region to take a 5-minute stroll (indoor song, fitness center, shopping center), try doing five mins of mild stretches at domestic.

For dinner, eat some component filling however slight:

•Herb and mushroom rice casserole

•Artichoke coronary coronary heart and bean salad

•Potato, leek, and bean soup

After dinner, set 10 to 15 mins apart for the Gratitude Meditation. The first few days of cleansing can be hard on the body and make you enjoy worse in some instances. It is important to offer manner to and do not forget what you need to be thankful for so you cognizance greater on gratitude and much less on what your frame is feeling. This can help save you you from forsaking the cleanse.

Day 2

Begin your day with a detoxifying beverage:

•Lemona (boosts electricity simply)

•Pomegranate and beet juice (boosts immune machine)

After your beverage, repair yourself a bowl of blended melon. Include any of the subsequent:

•Watermelon

•Honeydew

•Cantaloupe

•Muskmelon

Also, revel in a small part of cinnamon porridge collectively with your blended melon.

At lunchtime, address yourself to an antioxidant smoothie:

•Almond banana bread (suitable supply of antioxidants; potassium; vitamins A, C, and K; and a splendid source of omega-three fatty acids)

•Honey mint (complete of minerals like copper and magnesium, additionally true in opposition to seasonal allergic reactions)

To entire your lunch, add in an artichoke coronary coronary heart and bean salad.

In the afternoon, take another 5-minute walk out of doors, climate permitting. If the climate is terrible otherwise you do now not have a incredible indoor region for strolling, perform a little essential stretches or throw some music on and dance like no individual is searching out five to ten mins. Dancing freely may be pretty releasing in masses of methods!

With your dinner, drink a cup of dandelion tea with raw honey. Have yourself some Dijon salmon with steamed veggies and wild rice.

When your day is winding down, set aside 10 to 15 mins for every other Gratitude Meditation. Keeping your self in right spirits and focused on what you are grateful for will preserve to provide you the highbrow and emotional stability to push via the soreness of the number one few days of fasting and cleansing.

Day 3

Before ingesting breakfast, address yourself to a cleansing, detoxifying beverage:

•Cucumber-mint detox

•Orange, carrot, and ginger detox

For breakfast, have a bowl of berry and seed porridge.

At lunchtime, drink a cup of dandelion tea with the glowing-squeezed juice from a slice of lemon and some uncooked honey. Eat a cup of carrot and lentil soup with a sparkling apricot on the side and a handful of combined nuts and seeds.

Sometime amongst lunch and dinner, make time to take a ten- to 15-minute walk outside. This stroll need to no longer be excessive or rigorous. It is supposed to be a casual walk so you don't overextend your body or energy. While fasting and cleansing, you will probably experience dizzy or willing, however every day exercise remains vital. Take it gradual and don't overextend your self till you sense pain or cause harm. If the weather is awful, discover an indoor area to walk for 10 to fifteen mins.

Dinner at the 0.33 day can be olive basmati rice with a detoxifying "drink your veggies" fruit and vegetable juice.

Close your day enjoy with a 15-minute Mindfulness Meditation to help you reconnect along with your frame. At this factor, you'll be starting to come out of the lousy, crummy, nearly gradual feeling of the detox flush. Shifting your mentality to be extra related in your body goes to help you experience that changes are taking region so you can understand the development this software program is providing.

Day four

Start your day with a detoxifying flush beverage:

•Lemona

•Pomegranate and beet juice

For breakfast, revel in an antioxidant smoothie:

•Almond banana bread

•Smoothie verde (excessive in weight loss program C and exclusive essential nutrients)

With your smoothie, revel in a cup of crucial seed porridge.

For lunch, do this kind of cleansing salads:

•Salmon fillet salad

•Rainbow trout salad

•Anchovy salad

Drink a cup of detoxifying juice rich in nutrients, minerals, and antioxidants.

During the afternoon, set apart 10 to 15 mins for a stroll outside. If the climate isn't proper for an outdoor stroll, find out an indoor area. At this factor on your cleanse, power need to be returning. At the very least, your frame obtained't experience so susceptible anymore due to the fact it's miles adjusting to the cutting-edge meals and smaller quantities. If you need to take a greater practical walk, begin gradual and don't overdo it. You can start a strength strolling regime even as taking precautions against dehydration and overworking yourself.

Eat a moderate and filling meal for dinner:

•Rice-stuffed peppers with salad

•Super quinoa salad

With your dinner, drink a cup of dandelion tea flavored with raw honey and a spritz of glowing lemon juice from a slice of lemon.

To loosen up at the give up of your day, set 10 to fifteen minutes aside for the Deep Breathing Meditation. Keeping your breath robust and your frame vitalized with oxygen may additionally have a primary effect in your flush in conjunction with the growth in exercising.

Day five

To begin day 5 of your liver flush, enjoy a detoxifying beverage:

•Cucumber-mint detox

•Orange, carrot, and ginger detox

Have an apple or a pear with a handful of nuts and seeds. Drink a tumbler of "drink your veggies" cleansing juice collectively along with your breakfast.

At lunch, drink a cup of dandelion tea with raw honey and the sparkling lemon juice from one lemon slice.

For your meal, have every:

•Potato, leek, and bean soup

•Herb and mushroom rice casserole.

On the factor, eat a fruit salad made of blended melons and antioxidant-wealthy berries.

In the afternoon, take a fifteen-minute walk out of doors, weather allowing. Or locate an indoor location in which you could walk for 15 mins. If your energy ranges are up for it, keep on with power walking so you can decorate your metabolism and work in the direction of a wholesome frame weight.

For dinner, try this form of leafy, nutrition-rich, cleaning salads:

•Artichoke coronary coronary coronary heart and bean salad

•Rainbow trout salad

When you've finished dinner and are on the brink of wrap up your day, set 10 to fifteen mins apart for a meditation exercise. On your fifth day, you'll be returning to the Gratitude Meditation. Even despite the fact that your frame is being used to the modifications you've made for the flush, gratitude is a completely important mindset to foster, particularly in preserving up with and keeping your liver health long time.

Day 6

Begin your day with a flush beverage to detox:

•Lemona

•Pomegranate and beet juice

Enjoy one of the porridge alternatives for breakfast:

•Cinnamon porridge

•Berry and seed porridge

•Essential seed porridge

Also, address yourself to an antioxidant smoothie:

•Almond banana bread

•Honey mint

•Smoothie verde

For lunch, have a tumbler of sweet carrot fruit and vegetable juice (immoderate in vitamins, minerals, and antioxidants). Eat a bowl of blended melon at the side of a chickpea and sesame seed salad.

Before dinner and after lunch, make time to take a 15-minute stroll, preferably out of doors however internal if the weather isn't first-class. Stick to on foot, even if you want to quicken the pace a chunk. With any shape of fasting cleanse, it isn't advocated that you push your self to jog or run, even in case you feel like your strength levels are "lower again to normal." Part of a fasting cleanse is to lessen your caloric consumption, which means that that your frame obtained't be in a nation for extra tough exercise.

With your dinner, drink a cup of dandelion tea with a spritz of smooth lemon juice and some raw honey. Whip your self up a few Thai-style snapper for a delicious detox meal.

Relax with a 10- to 15-minute Deep Breathing Meditation to wrap up your day and gradual down your body, thoughts, and feelings.

Day 7

On the final day of your immoderate flush, start your day with a detoxifying beverage:

•Cucumber-mint detox

•Orange, carrot, and ginger detox

For breakfast, have a nice fruit salad with mixed berries, melons, and apples. Accompany your fruit salad with a handful of blended nuts and seeds.

At lunchtime, drink a cup of dandelion tea flavored with a bit of sparkling-squeezed lemon juice and raw honey. Eat a cup of soup for lunch:

•Carrot and lentil soup

•Potato, leek, and bean soup

Also, revel in a glowing apricot, mango, or kiwi together along with your soup.

Give yourself 20 mins amongst lunch and dinner to take a stroll outside. If the climate isn't excellent enough for an out of doors walk, discover someplace interior wherein you may have a nice 20-minute walk. Movement and blood glide are both crucial to health and detoxing. Both hold fluids and waste transferring thru your body till they will be removed. When you sweat, you launch pollution via your pores, and this is a superb manner to sincerely growth your power levels. Still stick with informal strolling or electricity strolling. You obtained't need to embark on a extra rigorous exercising plan till after your seven-day flush.

With your dinner, drink a tumbler of candy carrot juice. Eat one of the moderate-but-filling meal options:

•Super quinoa salad

•Rice-filled peppers with salad

•Dijon salmon with wild rice and steamed vegetables

When your day is winding down, do every one-of-a-kind 15 mins of Mindfulness Meditation to reconnect together together with your frame. You is probably amazed to look at adjustments due to the fact the very last time you in all likelihood did this meditation. Connecting collectively at the side of your body in this way enables you shape a more fit attachment and courting to your self and your physical frame, and that is going an prolonged way within the path of prolonged-term fitness and preserving health and well-being.

Three-Day Liver Rejuvenation

You did it! You made it through the seven-day intense liver fasting flush! At this factor in the utility, your liver has been given each week-extended damage from all the matters that can be consumed and purpose troubles for it. You can also be capable of sense crucial changes for your body as a protracted way as natural power stages, enhancements in temper, feelings of readability, and clearer pores and pores and skin. These are all brilliant accomplishments! Even if you could't see any number one adjustments, the clean truth which you made it via is a first rate accomplishment in its very own proper.

Now comes the three-day software program wherein you may be rehabbing your liver. This vital organ has been given a pleasant break. Now, it's time to remind it the way to feature in a healthy way and hold up with what is being established your frame. When it includes this rejuvenation duration, you'll need to paste to the identical suggestions of what to avoid as had been laid out within the above section.

A lot of the components, drinks, and standards are despite the fact that the identical during this 3-day duration. You don't need to carry again materials like alcohol, dairy, and meat in advance than your liver has a hazard to recharge and rejuvenate. You will, but, have extra leniency on the subject of including snacks, cakes, larger portions of food, or maybe terrific forms of workout into the rejuvenation approach. Your body and liver were flushed. Now it is time to get the liver once more on route.

For all 3 days, begin with a detoxifying beverage:

•Lemona

•Cucumber-mint detox

•Pomegranate and beet juice

•Orange, carrot, and ginger detox

For breakfast, experience an antioxidant smoothie:

•Almond banana bread

•Honey mint

•Smoothie verde

And one of the scrumptious, wholesome porridge alternatives:

•Cinnamon porridge

•Berry and seed porridge

•Essential seed porridge

After breakfast, provide yourself 10 to 15 mins for a brisk stroll, clean dance exercise, or exclusive mild exercise you can do in or spherical your house.

Allow yourself a midmorning snack of one of the following treats:

•Quinoa cups

•Hummus with olives and carrot sticks

•Mixed nuts and seeds

•Chia yogurt custard

Lunchtime is complete of severa opportunities. Have your self a glass of a detoxifying fruit and vegetable juice:

•Drink your veggies

•The detoxifier

•Sweet carrot

For your lunchtime meal, stick with a yummy form of salads:

•Chickpea and artichoke sauté

•Artichoke coronary coronary coronary heart and bean salad

•Super quinoa salad

•Salmon fillet salad

•Rainbow trout salad

•Anchovy salad

Between lunch and dinner, have another snack:

- Mixed melon

- Apple and carrot slices with almond butter

- Cashew coconut cookies

After your afternoon snack, deliver your self 30 to 60 minutes for a mild workout. This can be a jog, run, or taking over a yoga splendor, tai chi class, or unique guided software with a private teacher. You need to paste to slight exercise as your body stays rebuilding itself and its strength.

For dinner, enjoy a person of those delicious, mild, healthy, and filling meals:

- Herb and mushroom rice casserole

- Olive basmati rice

- Rice-stuffed peppers and a salad

- Dijon salmon with wild rice and steamed greens

- Thai-fashion snapper

- Carrot and lentil soup

- Potato, leek, and bean soup

With dinner, have a few other glass of one of the fruit and vegetable detox liquids:

- Drink your vegetables

- The detoxifier

- Sweet carrot

Don't overlook about dessert! Treat yourself to a tasty dessert along side:

- Pain perdu

- Baked stone give up result

- Rice pudding with clean berry topping

Remember to drink a cleaning cup of dandelion tea with uncooked honey and a spritz of sparkling-squeezed lemon juice.

As your day includes an stop, supply your self 10 to 15 mins to carry out the Gratitude

Meditation, Deep Breathing Meditation, or Mindfulness Meditation.

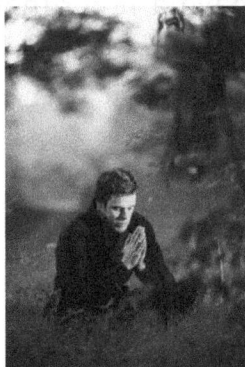

During this 3-day rejuvenation length, you've got got extra flexibility to mix and in shape what varieties of food you need to devour. You can mixture and healthful from the cleaning food and drink supplied, further to provide you together with your very personal. If you intend to make your very personal food and take a look at your very personal recipes, make sure that they adhere to the requirements of what to avoid, what to eat fairly, and what you could eat in abundance as laid out earlier than the seven-day flush breakdown.

Even even though the 3 days begin with 30 to 60 mins of mild exercise, you could even though want to ease into that so that you don't burn yourself out too early on. Exercise isn't in reality important to the cleaning, cleansing, and rejuvenating system. It is also going to help you with preserving a healthful weight and preserving your body in a mean extra healthy u . S .. Bodies that don't go together with the float and don't exercise are extra at risk of harm, infection, and disease, in spite of a wholesome liver. Give your self each advantage you may!

How to Use This Information and This Program

Use This Information for Your Own Health

Please don't forget that whilst you're making changes for your eating regimen, particularly inside the drastic way a flush begins offevolved, your frame goes to react. It isn't going to apprehend why its ordinary recurring changed so . This can reason sluggishness, fatigue, susceptible factor, dizziness, irritability, mood swings, and a sizeable crummy feeling.

Listen to what your body is telling you, but don't allow that crumminess deter you from intending with this machine. There is an adage that asserts "subjects need to get worse in advance than they get higher." In this example, your frame has to have time to adjust to the flush in advance than it'll begin cashing in on it.

That doesn't suggest there isn't a little room to make allowances. If you're suffering with the workout detail, perhaps great keep on with five or 10 mins of workout in preference to pushing for 15 or 20 mins. If you find out that your body cannot cope with the lower in power, offer yourself leeway to consume some of the snacks supplied within the Three-Day Liver

Rejuvenation section for the first couple days of your flush after which taper off. These allowances will assist your body modify more without troubles to the extreme detox.

If you undergo in mind it, the phrases detox, flush, and cleanse all advise some sort of drastic trade. Change isn't always smooth, and that is real for your body as nicely.

Detoxing regularly isn't advocated. Implementing the seven-day flush and three-day rejuvenation a part of this application isn't imagined to be completed every week or maybe each month. A cleanse paves the manner for a extra suit way of existence. It is as a good buy as you to hold your body and liver health among flushes via eating regimen, workout, and aware behavior.

When it involves weight reduction and retaining a wholesome weight, the very best technique for losing weight is to eat fewer energy than you burn every day. That is why fasting is a top notch manner to start this device. Our fasting software application reduces caloric consumption and promotes the burning of extra electricity through exercise and motion. If your body has been strolling tough to preserve a superb weight reputation that isn't your perfect weight, you would likely locate it even more difficult to make it thru the primary numerous days of the cleanse and detox. This is because of the fact your frame can nearly be bowled over by using manner of the short drop in caloric intake.

Be mindful of what your frame is telling you as a long way as your limits. In many times, together with in a cleaning snack that is absolutely low in energy is tons less risky to the flush plan than falling decrease returned to processed, unhealthy snacks to try to make yourself enjoy better.

A cleanse is meant to be extreme, however it isn't intended to make you sick or hurt you in any way. In some cases, humans with immoderate activities may in all likelihood benefit from starting with the 3-day rejuvenation utility to ease their frame into more wholesome foods, exercising, and reduce electricity earlier than stepping into the seven-day flush. If making a decision to keep in this way to save you your body and mind from experiencing surprise, undergo in mind to though observe the seven-day flush with a few different rejuvenation period. You can also want to tone down the workout portions if you don't get everyday workout.

A tip almost about cooking, meal prep, and fasting: If you want to maintain on time, you may constantly make a recipe that has multiple servings or double up on a recipe after which have the leftovers for lunch or dinner tomorrow/night time time. Be conscious that leftovers simplest maintain for a few days, so you'll need to be on pinnacle of consuming them or they'll visit waste.

When to Detox: How Often Should You Detox?

While there are not any set "guidelines" on how frequently or how seldom you need to detox, there are a few fitness issues. As formerly stated, detoxes and flushes aren't supposed to be a weekly or month-to-month event. Several individuals find that they favor to detox as quick as a 12 months, while others can also stick with or 3 times a 12 months. Then there are a few folks that will do it as soon as and be very strict in maintaining their health thereafter.

Truthfully, how regularly you want to detox is based totally on you and the way you experience. The exceptional advice we are capable of offer is to listen on your frame. You can exercise that with the conscious meditations that educate you to hook up with your body or via using continuing to hold your liver cleanse magazine whilst you entire the primary flush.

Whenever, or if ever, you acquire a issue in which your frame feels sluggish, you experience torpid, or the ones pre-cleanse signs and symptoms and signs and symptoms start to crop up all over again, that is probably an awesome time to do another cleanse.

Even in case you enjoy super all of the time, it's far impossible to preserve yourself loose from environmental pollution in our modern-day-day society. Air pollutants is one this is inescapable any time you step outdoor. That's no longer intended to discourage you from going outside because of the reality glowing air is also exquisite for fitness and nicely being. Environmental pollution maintain to pile up on your gadget irrespective of what lengths you take to hold your liver fitness.

With that in thoughts, a healthful aim is to try and detox three to four times a yr, every 3 or four months, specially in case you stay in a pollution-heavy environment, like vital metropolitan regions or places which have suffered from oil spills or special waste failures that have impacted the environment. Those toxic elements linger inside the environment for a long time.

Now that you have finished your flush, it's time to art work on preserving the fitness you have got were given have been given genuinely performed.

Chapter 5: How To Maintain A Healthy Liver

Doing a liver flush and detox is a first rate way to set up a healthful baseline for your liver. It receives rid of all of the poisonous junk that has built up on your frame and gives your liver a spoil. The flush is just one step to lengthy-time period liver health, even though. Once the liver is cleansed, in case you revert to the identical patterns and behavior as in advance than, that toxicity will sincerely build right decrease returned up another time.

One of the toughest elements of a wholesome liver and everyday health and properly being software is the protection. This may be difficult due to the fact renovation is prepared changing your manner of existence and making conscious, every day efforts to offer aid to your liver. Over time, these changes become a addiction. However, in the beginning, they may be difficult, mainly if they'll be properly outside of your pre-flush way of life.

True way of lifestyles modifications are a willpower. The suggestions in this financial ruin are going to provide you a solid foundation for constructing behavior that make and manual a satisfied liver. At this aspect, you may start to reintroduce dairy, meat, and eggs into your food regimen. Be aware that during moderation, the ones gadgets are excellent to eat. For lifelong liver health, regardless of the fact that, you'll need to in trendy devour meals and recipes that stick with the liver health and manual food that have been referred to in the previous bankruptcy.

Diet and exercising are of the primary components of maintaining health, in particular with regards to your liver. There are one of a kind self-care practices that you may start to artwork into your existence just so your frame and mind get a danger to lighten up and rejuvenate among cleanses and flushes.

Exercise

There are such a whole lot of options for exercise nowadays that the only actual hassle is finding the time. Unless you are a hardcore health buff, you only need 20 to 30 minutes of workout a day to hold your self. While forty five to 60 minutes of exercise a day is the encouraged minimum for health, it can be tough to discover that time every day with whole-time jobs, searching after a residence or a own family, having pets, and different responsibilities.

So, on the project of compressing workout in really for the purpose of having your frame moving, 20 to half-hour an afternoon can suffice. This exercising doesn't must be specially rigorous both. Taking a brisk, 30-minute walk in the nighttime to get your coronary coronary coronary heart fee up and blood flowing is a gentle exercise that keeps your body shifting and lets in beautify your metabolism.

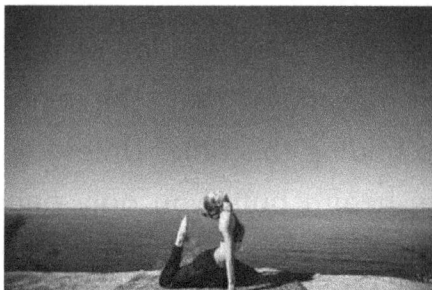

If you are crunched for time, a good tip is to look at exercising applications that you may do in your private home or spherical your private home. A 20-minute every day jog in your community can art work wonders to your body and metabolism. So can a 20-minute stretching everyday right on your private living room! Between YouTube and cell smartphone apps, there are masses of programs and films you can discover that train you inside the right manner to stretch.

Through those equal property, you could discover brief dancing workouts for health and packages like yoga, Pilates, and one-of-a-kind kinds of martial arts. All of those sporting events may be completed in your private home in an open vicinity. Just look for what you're inquisitive about on YouTube or your smartphone app keep, and you'll find out a plethora of wonderful topics and alternatives. A lot of those offerings are free too!

When the usage of apps and movies for at-home exercising training, search for the alternatives that deliver clear and unique instructions. If a stretch isn't performed efficaciously or a yoga position isn't held within the right manner, then it could stretch the wrong muscle or no longer provide the advantage that it is supposed to.

Exercising at home is a wonderful way to preserve time and money. It does require strength of will, motivation, and a willingness to analyze the proper actions, holds, stretches, and muscle use so that you don't inadvertently harm your self. There also are options for mild and moderate exercising that you can do out of doors the residence if you have the time and price range and feel like you could gain extra from proper guidance.

There are quite a few yoga studios spherical that provide splendid types of yoga and different varieties of exercise. You can do a brief search on your nearby place to find out yoga, Pilates, aerobics, tai chi, aikido, martial arts, and great classes that offer precise stages of exercise. You should even combo and in shape. Sign up for a yoga beauty more than one instances per week, and then persist with strolling or walking the relaxation of the week.

Please hold in mind that when you have weight reduction goals and fitness desires, you'll need to pursue a more installed, extreme workout regime. There is a difference amongst exercising for healthy motion and workout for fitness.

If your dreams are greater oriented inside the direction of weight reduction and building muscle tissues, then you'll need to bear in mind alternatives like a health club club. Gym memberships may be useful for human beings with tight schedules due to the fact there isn't a hard and fast time that you want to bypass. You can pass whenever you have the time.

Some gyms are even open 24 hours an afternoon now, so in case you want to head in in advance than or after paintings, they will be open.

Gyms provide the gain of various people working out, that could assist inspire you to exercising as well. A lot of gyms have non-public running shoes too. If you parent with a private trainer, they will assist teach you a way to drift and exercising well and assist you assemble an workout plan to satisfy your desires. A lot of gyms even have fitness instructions, just like a yoga studio, and participation is from time to time included in the gymnasium membership rate.

There are a few those who don't like exercise at gyms. Sometimes, having a health club club looks as if a excellent concept, and then it in no way gets used. Going to a gym does require motivation and self-management.

Also, a few humans find it uncomfortable to attempt running out or exercise spherical masses of various human beings, mainly if a number of the ones people are in a terrific deal better form.

While it isn't a competition approximately being healthy, this can but be hard.

If you're the type of character who doesn't need to go to a health club, you can even though discover extra excessive exercising commands or applications that have a specific surroundings. You can also enlarge a exercise normal at home with minimum system, together with precise weights, stretch bands with varying resistances, medication balls, and kettlebells.

During the seven-day flush and the 3-day comply with-up, you've got been recommended to encompass moderate to slight exercising into your every day everyday.

That modified into in an try to hold your body lively and help the detox method, but it have to not have pushed you beyond the thing of exertion on the equal time as your body come to be ingesting fewer strength.

When you begin forming a ordinary exercise regime for yourself as part of your maintenance manner of lifestyles, you'll need to ease into this device.

If you are new to ordinary exercising or have limited revel in, start gradual and progressively artwork up to a more hard, longer habitual. If you are an skilled exerciser however took a wreck in the course of your flush, then you absolutely definately'll although need to ease again into your regular. Your body is in a modern day usa of being, and it'll need the time to readjust so it is able to cope with that equal degree of intensity.

A few factors to keep in thoughts at the same time as exercise:

•Ease into it

•Learn the right manner to save you harm

•Take it gradual

•Find the technique or method that works for you and your life-style

•Don't stress it

•Gradually construct to your stamina and health

•Have fun

Massage and Self-Care

There is more to retaining health than in reality weight loss plan and workout. Self-care is one of the least referred to techniques for retaining your frame and mind wholesome. In a society that makes a speciality of taking walks extra difficult and being more effective, requirements like taking time to loosen up, rejuvenate, and do self-care are simply forged apart.

It is unfortunate, however you do have the ability to find out about self-care techniques that can gain you, your fitness, and your liver's health.

Massage

Some popular self-care sports activities encompass rubdown and spa services. Getting a massage isn't genuinely lying on a table and having your sore muscle organizations rubbed.

A lot of massage therapists art work to control the frame, getting rid of sources of continual ache, supporting reduce tension, and correcting frame posture that outcomes in pain and stiffness. During a rub down, loads of clients discover themselves in a totally cushty america wherein they aren't thinking about what to make for dinner, how many emails they need to reply at work, or the like.

They clearly get to reveal their mind off and enjoy the feeling of a healing touch.

Our society notably underestimates the strength of rest as a recovery method. In the case of rub down, whilst the conscious thoughts rests and the muscle mass, joints, and tissues of the body are manipulated through manner of using an out of doors supply, the inner techniques of the body have a hazard to "seize up." In the case of the liver, it has the danger to kick itself into tools on the identical time because the rest of the frame relaxes. It can growth its very personal functionality at some point of the rubdown.

By manipulating the muscles and joints of the body, rub down may be quite detoxifying in its very private right. It can get the metabolism going and loosen up muscle mass and tissues as a manner to release stored pollutants, letting them be nicely processed and removed.

Massage has turn out to be a favorite for pretty a few human beings, many who get massages as speedy as a month or maybe once each week because they get such extremely good highbrow and physical blessings from it.

There are even options to get couples massages for you and your accomplice or accomplice, or perhaps you and a chum, or with a little one, sibling, or decide.

Couples massages turn out to be imparting a nice fun surroundings for you and each one of a kind character, and they aren't unique to romantic relationships.

Massage isn't for every person, despite the fact that. Plus, it can get costly to have everyday massages. However, there are a few rub down strategies that you could learn how to carry out on yourself at

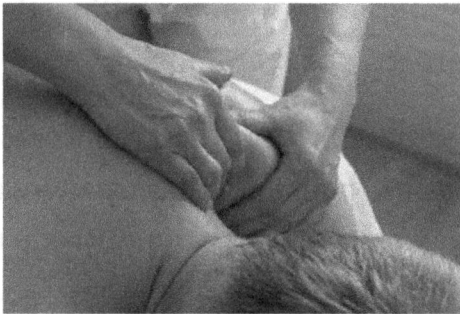

domestic which might be particularly geared inside the direction of releasing stagnant energy buildups in the course of the liver. Since your liver is connected to severa specific organs and frame structures, it is largely a superhighway of electricity.

This self-massage method will help preserve that electricity transferring fluidly, as a end result retaining the liver functioning healthily.

Liver Energy Stagnation Self-Massage

1.Scrunch your eyes closed tight, then open your eyes large. Repeat 30 times.

2.On your left hand, find the issue between your thumb and forefinger. It could be fleshy and a chunk mild if you press down on it. Gently draw near the factor among your right thumb and forefinger and perform a moderate, round movement with slight stress on that factor.

Complete 30 circular motions.

3.Repeat the above step for your proper hand.

4.Make a fist together collectively with your dominant hand, and beginning at the bottom of your throat, use the ridge of your knuckles to softly faucet down the center of your sternum. When you acquire the bottom of the breastbone, begin lower returned at the top. Repeat this movement 3o instances.

five.Place the heels of your fingers on the top of your belly muscular tissues and with mild to slight pressure, sink into your muscle businesses and push your hands down the period of your belly. In brushing strokes, repeat this movement at the center and facets of your abdomen 30 times.

6.Locate a issue immediately under the nipple inside the sixth intercostal place among the ribs. If you're a lady, that factor could be in which the underwire of your bra is or around the crease of your breast.

It might be a easy divot between the ribs. Gently press on that point on each components of the chest and do the spherical rubdown motion 30 times. Tip: If you could't locate the point precisely, use the flat fringe of your hand to do 30 from side to side strokes under the breast or pectoral crease to stimulate the element.

7.Repeat the belly massage step (Step 5).

eight.Using your hand to diploma the relativity in your body, maintain your pointer finger, center finger, ring finger, and pinky finger together so they may be flat and degree. Place the edge of your pointer finger at the base of your knee cap and use those 4 arms because of the reality the dimension distance to some extent for your shin. Once you have got the problem in your shin, trace a finger from the element to the outdoor of the shinbone, transferring to the outdoor of the leg. You'll discover a easy divot that is the acupressure factor you are searching out. Gently rubdown this thing in a circle 30 instances.

9.Repeat at the opportunity leg.

10. Using the equal finger measurement approach, begin with the sticking out ankle bone at the internal of your leg. Measure alongside the interior leg collectively together with your hands, and a few of the shinbone and calf muscle, you'll find out a tremendous, smooth divot. Gently rub

down this factor with a spherical massage motion 30 instances.

eleven. Repeat this step for your distinct leg.

12. With your pointer finger, discover the difficulty to your foot in which your first and 2d toe bones meet. Slowly slide your finger in advance until you find the clean dip a number of the 2 toes close to the pinnacle of your foot. In a round rubdown movement, lightly rubdown this point 30 instances.

thirteen. Repeat the identical step on the opposite foot.

The sort of round acupressure rubdown you are going to be doing is setting your thumb at the focused factors and doing mild, clockwise circles together collectively along with your thumb, with out eliminating the digit from the issue.

Spa Services

Spa offerings are each special famous self-care exercise. This doesn't without a doubt advise getting a pleasing nail decreasing or pedicure. Spa offerings encompass facials; body wraps; foot, hand, and face massages; or maybe head massages. There can be invigorating and exfoliating scrubs as well.

Such offerings can get costly; but, the techniques used are designed to be greater useful than definitely clearing pores and pores and pores and skin and making your hair, pores and pores and skin, and nails more aesthetically applicable. Some frame wraps and scrubs are designed to extract pollutants from within the frame. Others are designed to beautify the metabolism.

Some spas have offerings like infrared saunas which have precise sauna packages to help sell weight loss, pain comfort, and cleansing. While the sauna itself doesn't make the ones gadgets rise up, it allows set the proper wavelengths within the body just so at the identical time as you preserve on at the side of your exercise and healthy eating plan plans, they assist boom the famous outcome.

So, despite the fact that spa services are regularly taken into consideration a high-priced for rest, they can be pretty useful to the body in other methods. You might likely even recall growing a cleansing body wrap a part of your normal ordinary. While it gained't cast off the want for a whole-body flush, it is able to assist to stretch out the time in among cleanses and flushes.

Not to mention, spa services are typically pretty fun and may help repair your herbal electricity tiers. To make it even extra thrilling, see if you may get pals, family, or possibly your kids to join you for a spa day. It may be a notable social and bonding interest as nicely.

Mindfulness and Meditation

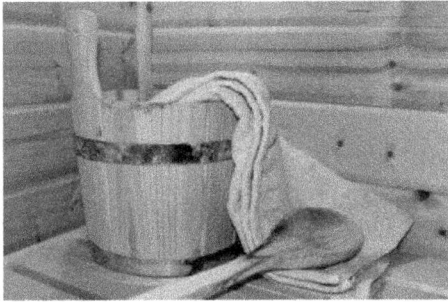

Although the spa services above are expensive, there are some self-care techniques you could put in force for yourself in your house. Meditation and mindfulness practices are very useful self-care packages that might beautify your each day lifestyles, health, and fitness.

If you are new to meditation and mindfulness, use the introductory meditations which is probably covered on this e-book that will help you via the seven-day flush. You can effects discover smartphone apps, YouTube movies, CDs, and podcasts that have guided meditations, commands on schooling meditation, and suggestions for conscious wearing occasions.

Since meditation is an workout for the thoughts, you'll have to ease into it, much like with body exercising. When you start, you possibly obtained't be capable of keep the meditation for more than 3 to five mins. After a while, that time gets longer. There are guided and group meditations which can ultimate for days!

Group meditations are every other way to enter the sector of meditation because of the fact you may talk your studies with a fixed and communicate to an trainer right now. Setting 10 to 15 mins aside a day for meditation can extensively enhance your concept styles and bring about bodily health and nicely-being as well as intellectual health and fitness.

It isn't quite much mastering to take a seat although, be quiet, and lighten up. There are many advantages to meditation and mindfulness workout, which encompass benefits to your physical health and your liver feature.

Self-Care Hobbies

A lot of talk approximately self-care manner that it's far intended to be some form of self-development whether or not or now not it's workout, a laugh, or converting concept patterns. The essence of self-care is ready making time for yourself and taking element in sports that provide you with strength and assist you to step faraway from your manner, your family, and your duties and experience some element for yourself.

Maybe you adore to read, however you haven't picked up a brand new ebook in years. Start studying yet again. Even if best for 10 or 20 minutes a day, make it a addiction and reconnect together at the side of your love of studying.

If you want gambling video video games, set a hint bit of time aside every day to play video video games. Generally, you don't need to pile on too much show display screen time due to the truth your eyes and thoughts want a break from all that blue slight. However, if gaming is your passion, make time for it.

Perhaps you don't have a hobby or ardour you love, but you've got typically desired to learn how to draw, knit, or throw horseshoes. Allow yourself the time to examine a new capacity, despite the fact that that capacity doesn't carry out a bit issue for your hobby, training, or normal existence responsibilities. The issue of self-care is giving your self a smash.

Even if those moves and interests don't especially pertain to liver fitness, they do contribute to prolonged-time period highbrow and physical health and nicely being. That prolonged-term fitness and well-being does encompass your liver as well. So, supply yourself some time and region every day for an hobby you want, some thing you're enthusiastic about, something it can be. Feed your self and nurture your self as an man or woman who isn't described via your duties. Your liver will love you for it!

Diet Tips for Maintaining a Healthy and Happy Liver

Even even though you've got got got superior beyond your seven-day flush, to keep proper liver fitness and decrease toxin buildup, you may want to live aware of what you're consuming and setting into your frame. When you aren't actively cleansing, you can deliver meat, eggs, and dairy once more into your food regimen. You may want to in all likelihood decide no longer to, and this is completely extraordinary as long as you are becoming wholesome stages of protein, minerals, nutrients, and probiotics through the rest of your weight-reduction plan.

Between flushes, you need to recollect the subsequent recommendations about your healthy dietweight-reduction plan and what's being positioned into your frame. Not only will they help manual your liver and its function, but they will assist make certain that the majority of toxin buildup is from environmental impacts.

Hydration

Fluids are one of the requirements to your body's functionality to smooth waste from your gadget. The kidneys and urinary device are waste filters, and that they require fluids to method waste. Most of the substances for your body that go along with the waft and flow into (e.G. Blood, lymph, and bile) are all fluids of some kind. So, imparting your frame with enough fluid to dispose of waste is important.

More than that, as your body tactics waste, it loses fluids. Your frame is prepared 60% water, so at the same time as it begins losing fluids for ordinary capability, it additionally begins offevolved to lose water.

Staying hydrated by using manner of eating hundreds of water goes to serve your body well.

It is also going to offer your liver with greater assist by using the usage of the usage of making the cleaning and flushing approach simpler as your liver techniques waste.

Caffeine

Caffeine is one of the most overused capsules in the global. Yes, it technically is a drug. No one thinks about it in that regard, even though.

Coffee and tea drinks are this form of regular part of day by day existence and society that a number of human beings can not make it via their day without more than one caffeine boosts.

The capture-22 is that relying on caffeine for electricity boosts impairs the body's capability to rely on its very very personal energy assets. Therefore, the whole body and body strategies emerge as more gradual, specifically if there isn't sufficient caffeine. This is one of the reasons why removing caffeine from the healthy dietweight-reduction plan all through a flush is so vital.

When you aren't actively flushing, you need to nevertheless don't forget moderating your caffeine consumption.

In terms of assisting lessen dehydration, limiting your coffee and tea intake to 2 cups an afternoon, 3 on the absolute most, is a remarkable concept.

Furthermore, caffeine has an exceedingly lengthy half of of-lifestyles, which means it remains inside the body for a long term. Sleep experts advocate not drinking any caffeinated liquids after approximately eleven a.M. So that the caffeine doesn't intervene with herbal sleep styles.

Sleep is some other vital feature for proper liver fitness. In fact, one of the signs of an unhappy liver is having sleep inconsistencies. Help your liver through helping your sleep and limiting your caffeine consumption.

Teaching your body to function to your herbal electricity levels is the healthiest method you could take.

Sometimes, it can be hard to choose yourself up in the morning and get to paintings with a clear thoughts. That is why caffeine is this sort of coveted substance. If you may end the dependancy and maintain on with your body's ordinary, natural, natural rhythm, you'll be surprised with the aid of the usage of how hundreds better you sense over time!

Avoid Alcohol

Alcohol is one of the maximum poisonous substances for the liver. It is every distinctive socially best drug that is quite abused, even via manner of individuals who aren't taken into consideration alcoholics. Any form of alcohol overuse is going to vicinity a strain on the liver.

Generally speakme, it's miles taken into consideration stable for women to have one alcoholic beverage an afternoon and for guys to have alcoholic beverages a day. Now, this doesn't suggest pour your self the most essential glass of wine you may and phone that one drink.

By dietary suggestions, the serving size for eighty-evidence liquor is 1.Five oz... A single serving length of beer is 12 ounces., and a single serving of wine is five oz..

What due to that is that pouring beers right right into a large glass despite the fact that counts as beverages. It furthermore approach that having a double shot of whiskey in a single glass still counts as drinks.

It is in reality well worth noting that those proportions aren't meant to be averaged over a given period. Say you drink seven beers every Saturday night time, however you then definately don't drink any alcohol for the relaxation of the week.

That doesn't balance out the alcohol consumption on that one night time time time. You despite the fact that substantially overtaxed your liver with the ones seven beers in a short duration.

Drinking alcohol has come to be a everyday, social hobby. Going to a bar with pals, bar hopping, and having beer and wine at a circle of relatives barbeque are taken into consideration regular.

If you're severe approximately searching after your liver and your extended-time period fitness, keep away from alcohol while you may. Be privy to what's considered "secure" alcohol consumption and avoid behavior like binge drinking.

Reduce Unhealthy Fats, Processed Foods, and Refined Sugars

Grocery stores are packed with substances that are whole of volatile fat, delicate sugars, and processed meals. In fact, most commercially offered products like crackers, chips, and meat have severa the ones dangerous additives.

The disadvantage is that eating too many horrific fat and delicate sugars can motive fatty liver sickness. This takes region even as the liver turns into clogged with fats buildup and can not characteristic as a clean out.

Try sticking to leaner cuts of meat and reducing away the fat trimmings in advance than cooking it. Meat in itself isn't typically dangerous, but the excess fats can cause troubles through the years. You might also additionally in reality have a take a look at ingesting grass-fed, loose-variety, and antibiotic-loose meats as nicely.

Processed meals are typically categorised as gadgets that come "pre-prepared." Crackers, chips, mac 'n cheese in a container, tortillas, and deli meats are examples of processed components. They consist of preservatives, and some of the dietary price is stripped away all through the food processing. Processed substances will be predisposed to encompass hidden sugars and excessive tiers of preservatives to boom their shelf lifestyles.

Preservatives can confuse the body into wondering that what it is eating is not food or nutritious.

Thus, the meals get processed as waste. Your body doesn't get the right nutrients, and your liver and filtration gadget are running time past regulation whenever you devour some element. Those hidden sugars increase over the years in a poisonous manner as properly.

Even fruit has higher concentrations of natural sugars. Fruit intake should be restrained to 2 or three portions an afternoon, and also you have to attempt to restrict or lessen out a few aspect else that includes diffused or delivered sugars.

For instance, preserve-offered peanut butter has sugar brought to it, together with a few volatile vegetable oils that translate into saturated and trans fats. You'd think peanut butter is just peanuts, but that isn't always how the food processing international works.

Organic, all-herbal, and uncooked foods are becoming more widely available and additional low value. While you don't need to go to the acute of consuming herbal and all-herbal, you can get more healthy, plenty much less processed food from natural and natural markets, farmer's markets, and the "all-herbal" meals sections in your grocery keep.

Eating out is a few distinct capacity manner to show your self to loads of terrible fat, sugars, and processed elements, especially if you're eating fast food. Sometimes, consuming out is extra to be had, or likely you are craving a few greasy French fries. There isn't always any problem with that, but recognize of ways often you're eating out. Moderation is the crucial component to stopping pollution from building up to your machine. Let your frame rest among your "eat outs" and provide your liver exact enough time to smooth up before consuming out again. If feasible, restriction your consuming out to a couple of times each week.

The recipes in this e-book are all crafted from uncooked, complete food materials. If you get inside the addiction of creating most of your food in that manner, you're already reducing manner once more on hidden sugars, dangerous fat, and preservatives. There is probably plenty of more recipe mind inside the final bankruptcy of this ebook to assist get you started out on filling your kitchen with elements, snacks, and food for you to gain your liver and assist lessen toxin buildup.

Avoid Paracetamol

Paracetamol is a commonplace painkiller that some human beings use each day. The liver is the number one organ for processing and filtering capsules. Not all drugs and drugs are immediately tough on the liver. However, paracetamol is a liver-hitting drug. If it's miles taken long time, it could motive liver harm.

As a preferred rule of thumb, taking no greater than four grams an afternoon (about 8 drugs or pills) for no greater than 3 consecutive days is considered steady. If you're experiencing sufficient pain to require greater doses or lengthy-term use, take a look at on the aspect of your doctor about options. While lengthy-time period medicine use will always take its toll at the frame and the liver, this unique medicinal drug is harsh for the liver to approach. Avoid it while you may, or ask your scientific doctor for alternatives.

Chapter 6: Can I Lose Weight With A Liver Cleanse Program?

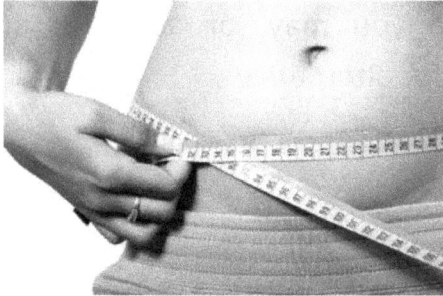

One of the most famous questions requested approximately liver detox packages is, can they help a person shed kilos? Weight loss is one of the most common motives why anybody should in all likelihood want to consider doing a software like a liver detox. It is actual that some of human beings battle to shed kilos with out suffering to benefit it. It is also real that a liver detox software program can assist in weight reduction.

As a natural filter for the body, it makes enjoy that the liver can assist to dispose of greater waste that could otherwise boom in the shape of adipose tissue, or fat tissue, in the body. Because our software puts an emphasis on motion and exercise in conjunction with enhancing liver characteristic and decreasing pollution inside the body, it will let you shed pounds. The kicker is which you want to understand how weight loss takes place. With that records, you may higher understand why a liver detox software program can help with weight reduction and a way to use it in your gain to attain your weight loss goals.

Before getting too concerned in liver detox and weight loss, permit's check a number of the commonplace misconceptions of weight reduction and notice why they may be misconceptions.

Debunking the Weight-Loss Myths

It is tough to discover reliable records approximately weight loss and weight-reduction plan nowadays. Everyone has a modern weight reduction tablet, a trendy "set up" diet, or a innovative manner to drop pounds in only some days. With that a tremendous deal records and that many hints flying round, how will you determine what is genuine and what works?

Getting back to the basics, if we have a examine weight loss in terms of weight loss plan and destroy it down into medical statistics, we ought to be capable of reduce via a number of the myths.

Calories

One of the maximum commonplace misconceptions approximately weight reduction is prepared counting power. This fable has carried out greater harm to weight reduction packages and regimes than a few different cutting-edge, newfangled diets.

Now, a calorie is simply an strength size. Each calorie consists of 4,184 Joules of power. This strength is what makes the body paintings as a complicated biochemical device.

Technically, the body isn't whatever more than a device, a supercomputer if you may, that completes biochemical techniques and runs off of strength. Every time you blink, beautify your arm, talk, form a idea, or explicit an emotion, your body is remodeling energy into movement or chemical tactics to result in the preferred final results. The frame doesn't sincerely make its very personal power, even though. In the same way that a slight desires a supply of electricity to expose on or a pc desires a battery or wire to plug into, the body dreams an electricity source.

For the human frame, that strength is energy. Calories come from the food we consume and the drinks we drink. On that foundation, it looks as if the body ought if you want to self-adjust. Feeling hungry on the same time as strength are strolling low, then feeling complete on the identical time as calories are fueled up. As the strength burn, that hunger feeling comes over again, almost like a automobile's tank of gasoline. When the tank gets low, you fill it up. Then it runs smoothly until the gas is burned up and the tank wants to be refilled. Your vehicle is in no way "overfull" of gas. How, then, does the body turn out to be "overfull" of electricity, main to weight gain?

Somewhere available can be the notion that 100 energy of spinach are identical to 100 energy of Oreo cookies. While the calorie amount is the identical, the manner the ones food are processed inside the frame isn't. Different kinds of sugars are metabolized thru the frame in wonderful ways. While a few sugars are transformed into electricity, others might be processed insufficiently, inflicting the calorie energy to be misplaced as extra warmness.

The one-of-a-type styles of food that you consume can effect the manner your body feels starvation. The thoughts and endocrine device produce hormones that manage starvation and ingesting behavior. If you are eating meals with micronutrients that stimulate the manufacturing of the hunger hormone, your frame will feel hungry, encouraging you to eat extra, even if you have ate up more strength than your body needs in a day.

Generally speaking, it's far considered healthy for ladies to devour among 1,six hundred and 2,400 strength a day. For person guys, the healthy caloric consumption is amongst 2,000 and 3,000. These numbers are in which the idea of "counting strength" as a manner to shed pounds is to be had in.

Unfortunately, it is extra complex than genuinely counting electricity. Not best are wonderful additives processed in a exclusive manner in the body, as cited above, but precise our our bodies require special caloric sustenance. For example, if you run 5 miles a day and are an person girl, you may consume greater electricity a day. To hold such an lively manner of existence and maintain your muscle tone good enough so that you don't injure yourself or turn out to be suffering with malnutrition, you need to top off the ones large portions of energy being burned.

On the flip factor, in case you paintings at a table 60 hours every week and the most exercising you get is walking to and from your vehicle to your administrative center or residence, then it's miles no longer going that you are burning very many power a day outside the minimal motion for calorie burning.

Exercise is only one difficulty to recall whilst energy are concerned. An man or woman who weighs more can burn greater energy walking one mile than an individual who weighs an awful lot much less. So, weight in itself is likewise a attention in how many electricity are being burned in correlation to how active you're.

Another difficulty in the back of calorie burning is genetics. There are some genetic predispositions which might be going to contribute to whether or not or now not your body can maintain up with burning the calories which can be fed on.

Considering the metabolic pathways, how one-of-a-kind meals are processed, and the quantity of exercise and modern-day weight, you can see that there are masses of methods strength can be processed and burned. This manner that no longer all power are created equal, so to talk. Thus, in reality counting strength isn't going to be enough to shed pounds.

Another important be privy to energy and counting energy. It isn't quite loads the styles of sugars and substances which you are consuming. It is also about what is in the ones ingredients. For instance, mainly processed meals and elements with preservatives are plenty more hard for the body to digest and destroy down into vitamins. This is mostly a give up stop end result of the factors and compounds no longer being absolutely recognized as "food" or "nutrients" through the body. As a end result, preservative-heavy meals can motive distinctive troubles that cause weight advantage.

Foods that take longer to machine and digest can cause the frame feeling hungrier due to the fact nutrients have now not been processed and absorbed. You may also turn out to be ingesting greater due to the fact the digestive device is burdened about what it is trying to interrupt down. Additionally, if the digestive machine doesn't recognize a manner to approach remarkable preservative-heavy components, then in desire to translating the meals into nutrients and caloric strength, they might get processed as waste. If big portions of meals are being processed as waste, the liver and extraordinary filtration structures can get backed up, and that waste builds up as frame fat. This additionally technique that you might be counting energy religiously, however in case you're however eating junk food and quite processed meals, you received't see an development in weight reduction.

Once that system is subsidized up, it can't seize up if the equal exceptional and portions of meals are being ate up regularly. It just offers to the problem. Going decrease lower back to hunger and the body being a machine, while extra weight starts amassing in the body, it turns into a far much less electricity-inexperienced machine. What which means is more energy is wanted to run the device.

Consider this: Eating 500 power of a meals like ice cream, cookies, or cake might be very clean. These are excessive-calorie additives. Trying to devour 500 power of spinach, carrots, or bananas could grow to be masses greater tough. This is a terrific example of techniques first-rate substances impact the weight loss system. Eating 500 strength of cake is simple and possibly wouldn't leave you feeling complete. In assessment, you may must strain your self to devour 500 calories of carrots, and also you'd be too complete to complete.

As for a body, humans with greater body weight will be inclined to eat massive portions or sense hungry extra often. This is due to the fact the frame desires extra electricity to keep its big mass. This is a few specific motive dropping weight may be tough due to the reality the urge to eat extra is a forestall give up end result of gaining weight and additionally hinders weight loss.

Exercise

Another myth approximately dropping weight is that eating regimen is enough.

There are hundreds of food regimen programs available advertising and marketing low energy, low carbs, no introduced sugar, and such a number of specific attractive ideas that delve into the generation about how counting carbs can help shed pounds. Unfortunately, masses of those applications gloss over one essential flaw. Diet on my own isn't sufficient.

The exquisite actual equation you want to understand in phrases of weight loss is that in case you constantly burn greater electricity than you devour, you'll shed pounds. When you consume tons plenty less and burn extra, your body starts offevolved offevolved to burn away more stores inside the shape of adipose tissue and body fat to make up for the lower amount of consumed strength.

To hold to maintain your dietary desires (now not venturing into unstable consuming habits that might cause eating troubles) on the equal time as additionally burning enough strength to begin dropping weight, growth your amount of exercise.

The time period exercise often comes with the stigma of lengthy exercising exercises, heavy sweating, and being in a gymnasium lifting weights. The splendor of exercise, although, is that motion is largely exercising. If you're committed to dropping weight, you'll likely must have a look at more rigorous exercising plans. However, depending on the quantity you need to lose, or if you are genuinely searching for to hold your weight, you don't need to move the complete nine yards.

There are plenty of moderate and mild workout options that, at the same time as mixed with extra healthful eating and liver cleansing, can assist in the weight reduction way. Exercise is ready extra than simply burning strength, though. Exercise stimulates your metabolism. This approach that your digestive machine is on foot greater correctly. It moreover enables to remove pollutants from your frame that is probably hindering fats burning.

It is critical to well known that, at the same time as the liver detox and 7-day flush can set your frame up to begin losing weight, it is absolutely one step of the gadget. This is why our seven-day cleanse software consists of slight exercising. Not pleasant is it going to initiate weight reduction inside the route of the flush, but it's also going to help you to get into the routine of gentle to slight exercising.

Our reason is to offer you what you need for success together along with your liver, extended-term fitness, and weight reduction dreams. That is why we've committed a whole financial ruin to weight loss via the liver detox application.

Another component of workout you will possibly word is that, in case you are actively losing weight, you would possibly grade by grade want to boom the time frame or intensity that you are exercise for. As you shed pounds, your frame goes to want greater exercise to burn extra power. Once you hit a aim weight, you could drop back off to maintaining that weight with slight or mild exercising if that is your desire.

The delusion approximately workout and weight reduction is that it isn't critical for weight loss. Truthfully, workout is fairly essential for weight loss. Both workout and diet plan play essential roles in weight loss and keeping weight. What it comes right down to is balancing weight-reduction plan and exercise.

One note about weight loss to consider is that from time to time as you workout, you may lose frame mass and adipose tissue, however you may not always see a big drop in weight. One of the reasons this will arise is that muscle mass is denser than adipose tissue. As you lose adipose tissue and benefit muscle groups, the exchange-off might not equal out to a huge drop in weight. If you're experiencing this phenomenon, bear in mind monitoring muscle tone development in addition to shrinking body mass in regions that have been as an alternative riddled with adipose tissue.

Low-Carb Vs. High-Protein Vs. Low-Fat Diets

Some of the maximum commonplace weight loss diets which may be all of the rage encompass excessive-protein diets, low-fat diets, and coffee-carb diets. Each of these diets has taken into consideration considered one of a kind motives for why they'll be advertised as being a achievement.

Taking a examine the excessive-protein diet, it is regularly advertised as growing the body's metabolism. This is the myth of the protein eating regimen. Honestly, the purpose the excessive-protein food regimen can paintings is that it shrinks the urge for meals. Protein is a filling micronutrient, taken into consideration the maximum filling. When you boom your protein intake, you experience a good deal less hungry; as a result, you consume fewer calories throughout the day.

One of the upsides to a excessive-protein healthy dietweight-reduction plan includes losing weight without counting energy. By developing your protein intake, you're putting fats loss on autopilot. Studies have shown that folks that prolonged their protein consumption to 30% of their each day energy started out out to unconsciously devour over four hundred fewer energy a day and out of place as a bargain as 11 pounds in 12 weeks (Gunnars, 2018, para 35).

Protein requires the body to use extra power to metabolize it. Thus, the excessive-protein diets burn fats due to the truth they expend extra strength virtually to be processed inside the body.

For almost decades, there were discrepancies the various low-carb and espresso-fats diets. Getting down to the nitty-gritty, low-carb diets do result in a lower caloric consumption than a low-fats healthy eating plan. It has been found out via consistent checking out that low-carb diets can growth weight loss two to a few instances more than low-fat diets (Gunnars, 2018, para 48).

As a state-of-the-art rule, low-carb diets reduce common urge for food. As with the excessive-protein eating regimen, a reduced urge for meals results in a reduced caloric intake. The low-fats weight-reduction plan doesn't have the same benefit. Low-carb diets additionally will be predisposed to drop water weight and reduce bloating in the body. This consequences in a substantial distinction in weight reduction as properly.

Eating a low-carb diet plan usually results in higher protein consumption as well. Therefore, the excessive-protein food plan benefits work at the side of the low-carb advantages.

If you've had any questions or troubles approximately strength, exercising, and the brilliant weight loss diets to be had, hopefully, the ones questions have been spoke back. Using the data above, the following section will discuss how our liver detox application permits with weight reduction.

How the Liver Detox Program Will Help You Lose Weight

Considering the facts above, one of the components of the seven-day liver flush is sticking to a low-calorie food plan. Not only is your caloric intake decrease because of the truth that fasting is a component, but the meals you are consuming are also all entire, uncooked factors. That technique they aren't very processed and aren't excessive in preservatives.

Those mixed characteristics imply that your body may also have greater ease digesting them and additionally in transforming them into vitamins and energy. Fewer fat, sugars, and processed chemical substances will building up on your machine as pollutants left over from improperly digested food.

Additionally, a fasting plan, on the facet of the low-calorie nature of the flush, will help reduce water weight on your frame. Any additional bloating or more water may be used up and removed. A as an alternative huge style of human beings stay in an nearly regular nation of bloating. This is often due to an overconsumption of processed grains and dairy. There are elements that boom extra water and inspire the frame to keep onto it.

By following the seven-day liver detox, you substantially reduce down on water weight, that could result in substantial weight reduction. It is proper to take away that water weight, and as a cease end result, you may enjoy lighter, have extra power, and enjoy extra bodily in shape.

One of the signs and symptoms and symptoms of a gradual liver is surprising weight gain. The liver also can get clogged with horrible fat fed on via meals. As such, it may't clear out fats out of the body nicely. This effects in unexpected weight advantage. By finishing a liver detox, you rid your body of pollution and those fats buildups. This gives your liver the danger to begin strolling at entire velocity over again.

When the liver is on foot at whole velocity, it could help keep the stableness among calorie processing and weight advantage. It additionally permits the digestive tool to hold shifting substances thru the method of being damaged down and can help clear out the waste that is available in an entire lot tons much less wholesome elements.

By following the renovation guidelines for lengthy-term liver fitness, you set up a healthy machine to your body that permits your liver to better keep the famous weight in amongst cleanses. More than that, a healthful liver will prevent surprising weight benefit. Seeing as that could be a signal of an dangerous liver, it stands to motive that the opportunity is actual of a healthful liver.

Keeping in thoughts that a healthy dietweight-reduction plan isn't sufficient to inspire huge weight reduction, take into account that an amazing detox program encourages an exercising recurring in order that it could maximize weight reduction and weight management.

Detox Programs Aid in Physical Movement Improvement and Physical Strength

As a biochemical system, the frame calls for a superb amount of lubrication to function. Think of an engine wanting oil or gears wanting to be greased to keep turning. There are a few structures inside the frame that don't have an organ much like the coronary heart to pump the vital fluids through the frame. The lymphatic device is one such device. Lymph additionally contributes to a healthy immune system and aids in waste removal.

When the frame is entire of pollutants, it turns into sluggish. This sluggishness also can take place as stiff joints. Sodium builds up, fats builds up, and bloating and swelling can get up whilst the liver isn't functioning nicely or if it's miles sluggish and blocked. Those buildups bring about sluggishness and lethargy.

These buildups can also reason an ordinary crummy feeling. When you enjoy that gradual and torpid, it's miles difficult to have the strength or motivation to exercising. Toxins within the frame can purpose a number of numerous troubles, on the aspect of trouble with motion.

Since a detox software gets rid of toxin buildup from the frame, it moreover will growth your electricity reserves so you can take a walk, bypass for a jog, or visit the health club and feature higher movement.

Flushes and detoxes moreover help to beautify electricity and muscle tone. As you detox, you lose adipose tissue. Your body becomes leaner and extra energetic. When you start to workout more, your leaner frame will construct strength and muscle quicker. The more your bodily form improves, the much less hard it'll be to preserve your desired weight.

Chapter 7: Why Is The Liver Important?

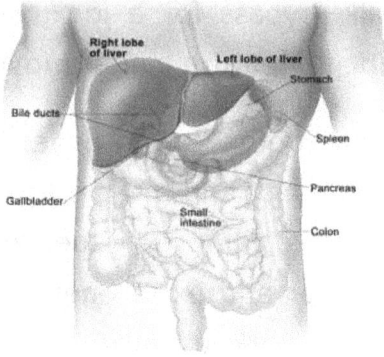

The liver is the body's largest internal organ. It weighs in at 3 kilos (1.Four kg.). The liver constantly holds round 13% of the body's blood at any given time. This is due to the fact a number of the blood from exclusive organs ought to bypass via the liver for severa techniques.

It is predicted that the liver has extra than 500 vital talents. Some of these embody helping in the digestive approach, metabolizing carbohydrate, lipids, and proteins, storing vitamins, detoxifying the frame, and supplying immunity for the frame to fight contamination and illness. Its characteristic is so vital that when it fails tissues in the route of the body can die off rapid from the lack of electricity and nutrients that the liver usually gives.

WHAT ARE THE FUNCTIONS OF THE LIVER?

DIGESTION

All the blood that leaves the belly and intestines passes thru the liver. The liver strategies the blood and breaks down the vitamins into paperwork which might be much less complex for the body to use.

The liver active feature in the method of digestion includes the manufacturing of bile. Bile is a fluid this is made and launched with the resource of way of the liver, but is saved inside the gallbladder. It breaks down massive clumps of fats into fatty acids, that would then be taken into the frame by way of the use of the digestive tract. One of the number one veins inside the liver, the hepatic duct, transports the bile produced with the aid of the usage of the liver to the gallbladder. During digestion of a meal, the muscular tissues within the walls of the gallbladder settlement to push bile into the bile ducts that result in the duodenum (first a part of the small gut). Once within the duodenum, bile allows with the digestion of fats. The liver, gallbladder and exceptional organs work collectively to digest our meals into its most simple building blocks.

METABOLISM

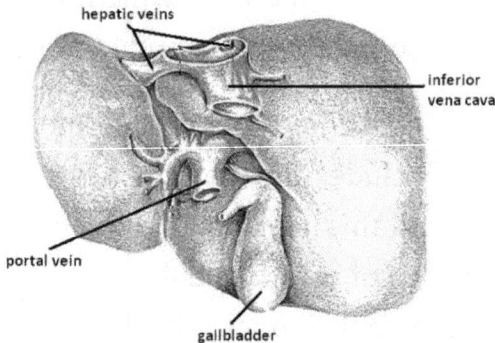

hepatic veins

inferior vena cava

portal vein

gallbladder

The liver performs an vital role in regulating your metabolism. This is due to the reality it is responsible for max of the chemical degrees to your blood. It takes the easy building blocks of meals (amino acids) and synthesizes complex substances from the additives (proteins). The production of protein is important for building the additives of your frame, which consist of muscles and bones. Protein moreover allows to stability your PH tiers and growth your immunity.

Ammonia is a derivative of this amino acid to protein technique. The liver breaks down this poisonous substance right proper right into a milder complicated known as urea, that is then launched into the blood. Urea then travels via the bloodstream to the kidneys and is exceeded out of the frame in urine.

The liver plays a principle role within the synthesis of glucose too. The liver breaks down carbohydrates into glucose for the body to use. Glucose is the primary sugar that is the precept power deliver for the body.

It is also the place of producing for pink blood cells in the first trimester of fetal development. Finally, the liver is likewise liable for the manufacturing of severa vital protein components of blood plasma accountable for blood clotting.

STORAGE

The liver is liable for regulating your blood glucose degrees. When you consume a

meal, the liver senses the growth to your blood sugar degree and eliminates sugar from the blood and stores it for use later, inside the shape of glycogen. Later, while you are hungry and your blood sugar stages are low, the liver breaks down glycogen and releases sugar into the blood.

 The liver does now not best store sugar, but minerals, which embody iron and copper too. Vitamins A, D, E, K, B12 and folic acid all stay in the liver too.

DETOXIFICATION

The liver acts like a blood filter out for the frame, walking hard to put off undesirable materials from the bloodstream. When the liver well-knownshows this form of pollutants, it

 breaks it down and removes it, each via the urine or feces.

Bile with the aid of-merchandise, alongside facet pollution in food, input the intestine and in the end leave the frame in the form of feces. Blood via-merchandise, consisting of drug remedies, are filtered out through using the kidneys, and go away the body within the shape of urine.

Another important feature of the liver includes the removal of bilirubin. Bilirubin is a continual substance that remains inside the returned of at the same time as new blood cells replace antique blood cells. The liver permits to interrupt down bilirubin and it is then voided thru your stools.

IMMUNITY

The liver is the powerhouse of your immune machine. The fundamental motive for this is because of the reality the liver homes Kupffer cells, which clean massive volumes of blood right away and efficaciously.

These cells have receptors on their floor that enjoy poisonous rely. The cells engulf and breakdown toxic count collectively with microorganisms, bacteria, fungi, parasites, tired blood cells, and mobile debris. Kupffer cells deal with this toxic rely with the aid of truly digesting it until it becomes a miles more stable substance.

The liver is likewise domestic to herbal killer (NK) and natural killer T (NKT) cells, which might be part of the innate immune tool. These killer cells modulate liver harm due to the truth they're anti inflammatory. Studies have shown that the ones cells play important roles in antiviral and antitumor defenses and inside the pathogenesis of chronic liver illness.